LUMBAR SPINE DISORDERS

Current Concepts

Volume 2

LUMBAR SPINE DISORDERS

Current Concepts
Volume 2

Editors

R. M. Aspden
R. W. Porter

Department of Orthopaedic Surgery
University of Aberdeen

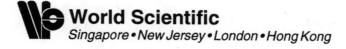

World Scientific
Singapore • New Jersey • London • Hong Kong

Published by

World Scientific Publishing Co. Pte. Ltd.
P O Box 128, Farrer Road, Singapore 912805
USA office: Suite 1B, 1060 Main Street, River Edge, NJ 07661
UK office: 57 Shelton Street, Covent Garden, London WC2H 9HE

British Library Cataloguing-in-Publication Data
A catalogue record for this book is available from the British Library.

LUMBAR SPINE DISORDERS: CURRENT CONCEPTS, Vol. 2

ISBN 981-02-2792-2

Printed in Singapore.

The fear of the Lord is the beginning of wisdom

Psalm 111

Motto of the University of Aberdeen,
which celebrated its quincentenary in 1995

CONTENTS

ACKNOWLEDGEMENTS

We gratefully acknowledge the support of Action Research who enabled the University of Aberdeen to establish the Sir Harry Platt Chair of Orthopaedic Surgery and the academic Department of Orthopaedic Surgery. We would also like to thank the Arthritis and Rheumatism Council, the Wellcome Trust, the Colt Foundation, the Sir Jules Thorn Charitable Trust and the National Back Pain Association who have funded our spine research in the Department.

PREFACE

This volume forms the second part of an anniversary book on 'Back Pain' to celebrate the quincentenary of Aberdeen University. In 1495 Bishop Elphinstone won the support of King James IV to provide a centre of learning in the North. Besides a University which would produce priests, schoolmasters and lawyers, James, who dabbled in medicine, may well have been Elphinstone's encourager to provide for the teaching of medicine and surgery. Playing to the remoteness of northern Scotland, he suggested that the inhabitants were "rude, ignorant of letters, almost barbarians" and were worthy of Britain's first medical school.

Now the capital oil-city of Europe, Aberdeen boasts of a prosperous economy, and a thriving University. 1995 also celebrated another anniversary - the fifth year of the founding of the University Department of Orthopaedics. Our strong interest in disorders of the lumbar spine prompted us to compile an anniversary book on "Back Pain Disorders", inviting contributions from friends around the UK who have done valuable research in this area. The tight schedule and the commitments of busy people meant that many potentially valuable contributions could not be included in the first volume, hence this second volume. Again, we have invited friends from many disciplines, basic scientists, physicians and surgeons, to share the results of their research on the most common of medical disorders. The outcome is deliberately personal and no attempt has been made to reconcile the differing views presented. This is meant to be provocative and reflects both the extent of our ignorance and the amount of active work that is still in progress.

One might ask why has back pain disability increased three fold in the past twenty years, when it has been the subject of so much excellent research? We know so much more about the structure of the spine, its physiology, and pathological change. We understand how discs become degenerate, and the complex changes that take place with neurological compromise. We have improved clinical skills, and better imaging. Our therapy is more refined. Surgical skills have improved, helped by impressive implant technology. Why then is back pain disability getting worse?

It is hardly possible that the environment is to blame. With such interest in ergonomics, the creation of a safe environment, and regulations on safe work handling, backs can not be suffering from greater mechanical stresses. Nor is it likely that in the workplace we now have a cohort of individuals with particularly weak backs. For the cause of increased disability we must focus rather on society and the socio-economic climate. This is beyond our immediate remit, but might be an area of productive research for a millennial volume. However enjoy the science, and muse on the answers to a major health problem. Perhaps we are still "rude, ignorant of letters, and almost barbarians".

CONTRIBUTORS

Robert Allen, PhD, CEng, FIEE, FIMechE, FIPEMB
Senior Lecturer
Department of Mechanical Engineering,
University of Southampton,
Highfield,
Southampton,
SO9 5NH

Alan Breen, DC, PhD
Research Director
Anglo-European College of
Chiropractic,
13-15 Parkwood Road,
Bournemouth,
Dorset. BH5 2DF

K. Bush, MB BS, MD(Lond)
Consultant Orthopaedic Physician
6 Harley Street,
London W1N 1AA.

P.R. Croft
Professor of Epidemiology
University of Keele
Industrial and Community Health
Research Centre,
North Staffs Medical Institute,
Hartshill Road,
Stoke on Trent, ST5 5BG.

H.V. Crock, AO, MD, MS, FRCS, FRACS
Consultant Spinal Surgeon
Cromwell Hospital
Cromwell Road
London SW5 0TU

Matthew Dolman, MB BS
Compass Junior Research Fellow
Bath and Wessex Orthopaedic Research
Unit,
Wolfson Centre,
Royal United Hospital,
Combe Park,
Bath, BA1 3NG.

J.C.T. Fairbank, MD, FRCS
Consultant Orthopaedic Surgeon
Nuffield Orthopaedic Centre,
Oxford, OX3 7LD.

H. Frost, MSc, MCSP
Director of Physiotherapy Research
Nuffield Orthopaedic Centre,
Oxford, OX3 7LD.

A. Garrett
Research Fellow
Department of Health Sciences
University of York
Alcuin College
Heslington
York, YO1 5DD.

S.P.F. Hughes, MS, FRCSEd(Orth), FRCS, FRCSI
Orthopaedic Surgery Unit,
Royal Postgraduate Medical School,
Hammersmith Hospital,
London W12 0NN.

J.R. Johnson, FRCS
Consultant Orthopaedic Surgeon
Princess Grace Hospital,
42-52 Nottingham Place,
London W1M 3FD.

M.R.K. Karpinski, FRCS, FRCSEd,
MCh (Orth), FRCSEd (Orth)
Consultant Orthopaedic Surgeon
Castle Hill Hospital,
Cottingham,
North Humberside, HU16 5JQ.

I.D. McCarthy
Orthopaedic Surgery Unit,
Royal Postgraduate Medical School,
Hammersmith Hospital,
London W12 0NN.

P.W. McCarthy, PhD
Senior Lecturer
Anglo-European College of
Chiropractic
Parkwood Road
Bournemouth, BH5 2DF.

S. Matsuda, MD
Cromwell Hospital
Cromwell Road
London SW5 0TU

R.C. Mulholland, FRCS
Special Professor in Orthopaedic
and Accident Surgery
34 Regent Street,
Nottingham, NG1 5BT.

J.E. Nixon, MA, ChM, FRCS
Consultant Orthopaedic Surgeon
King's College Hospital,
London SE5 9RS.

R.W. Porter, MD, FRCS, FRCSEd
Director of Education and Training
Royal College of Surgeons of
Edinburgh,
Nicolson Street,
Edinburgh EH8 9DW.

I.L.H. Reichert
Orthopaedic Surgery Unit,
Royal Postgraduate Medical School,
Hammersmith Hospital,
London W12 0NN.

Alistair Ross, FRCS
Consultant Orthopaedic Surgeon
and Director
Bath and Wessex Orthopaedic Research
Unit,
Wolfson Centre,
Royal United Hospital,
Combe Park,
Bath, BA1 3NG.

D. Ruta
Consultant
Department of Public Health
Tayside Health Board

F.W. Smith, MD, FRCPEd
Consultant in Nuclear Medicine
Aberdeen Royal Hospitals Trust,
Foresterhill,
Aberdeen, AB25 2ZD

P. Thorpe, FRCS, MRAD
Senior Registrar in Radiology
Aberdeen Royal Hospitals Trust,
Foresterhill,
Aberdeen, AB25 2ZD

J. Wilson-Macdonald, ChM, FRCS
Consultant Orthopaedic Surgeon
Nuffield Orthopaedic Centre,
Oxford, OX3 7LD.

CHAPTER 1

EPIDEMIOLOGY OF LOW BACK PAIN: THE BRITISH CONTRIBUTION

P.R. Croft

1. Introduction

The usual style of introduction to epidemiological studies in low back pain is an emphasis on the meagre supply of such investigations in the literature. This provides a helpful springboard for the authors to convince their readers that their own study is a novel and original contribution to an infant genre. There must come a time however when a critical mass of papers on the topic will have seen the light of publishing day, and such statements can no longer be maintained with tongue kept at a distance from cheek. Have we arrived there yet? In relative terms, the answer is certainly 'no', since compared with cancer or cardiovascular epidemiology, the field of back pain has a slender output. Yet there is now a body of work that is sufficient to review, even if as yet it provides only a limited exploration of most important issues related to the occurrence, causes and prevention of back pain in the community.

2. Why epidemiology?

Epidemiology traditionally has three concerns:

(i) describing and measuring the distribution of disease in populations
(ii) investigating what might cause or influence such patterns of occurrence
(iii) evaluating the outcome of interventions designed to prevent the disease or to reduce its impact

In the field of back pain there is now a solid body of evidence about its frequency and impact in the general population. There has been a distinctive British contribution to this, and the first part of this chapter will summarise it. This includes the extent of restrictions which back pain imposes on everyday living, its social impact, and the utilisation of health care by back pain sufferers. These are important issues in themselves, but are of specific relevance to epidemiological studies of back pain. This is because back pain does not kill people very often, and its occurrence and impact must be measured in some way other than mortality.

There are fewer epidemiological investigations of causes of back pain in comparison with the number of descriptive population studies. However there have been some British contributions to consider. There have also been clinical epidemiological studies concerned with issues of diagnosis and investigation and the extent to which epidemiological studies should be concerned with the 'back' and the 'spine' or with 'pain' as a focus of attention.

There is a growing literature of scientific evaluation of interventions to treat back pain. The process of assessing and integrating all these studies has begun, and some clues are beginning to emerge, with some distinctive British contributions. These have been considered in other chapters, but their potential impact on the occurrence of low back pain will be briefly considered here.

3. How common is low back pain?

The usual response to this question is to reply "It all depends on what you mean by low back pain". A major problem that affected the comparative epidemiology of low back pain for decades was that each new study chose its own distinctive definition.

Often the evidence was provided from large surveys which did not necessarily have low back pain as the focus of attention and relied on single unqualified questions for prevalence estimates. The Health and Lifestyle Survey for example was a large survey of some 9,000 British adults conducted in 1983[1]. A single question about current back trouble ("back problems in the past month") was included in the interview schedule, providing an estimate of the prevalence of low back trouble in the adult British population of 19%.

The classic surveys carried out by the Field Survey Unit of the Arthritis and Rheumatism Council (then known as the Empire Rheumatism Council) in the North West of England in the 1950's had the musculoskeletal diseases as their principal focus of attention. However the questions about back pain were still nonspecific. In these studies the estimated prevalence of low back pain in adults on the day of interview was 15%[2].

Publications in recent years have provided a more solid basis for prevalence estimates[3,4,5]. Such estimates remain firmly based on self-reported pain, a symptom rather than an objective sign or a finding that can be validated against some external criterion. These studies have a number of advantages over the earlier surveys. They were based on methods which defined what is meant by 'low back', specified the period of time to which the questions about symptoms apply, and introduced a variety of methods by which the low back pain can be classified, either based on pain characteristics (such as its severity) or on the restrictions of daily living to which the condition can give rise.

In 1991 Walsh and colleagues from the Medical Research Council's Environmental Epidemiology Unit in Southampton reported a study of 1172 men and 1495 women aged 20 to 59 years from eight areas in Britain[3]. Their sampling frame consisted of the age-sex registers of general practitioners in the seven towns and one rural district where the study was performed. The method employed was a cross-sectional postal survey. Low back pain was defined by a pre-shaded area on a mannikin or pain drawing, bounded by the twelfth ribs above and the gluteal folds below.

There were two separate definitions of time period in this study - pain during the year immediately prior to the survey, and pain 'ever'. Patients were asked to exclude menstrual pain, pain occurring during a feverish illness and pain during pregnancy. The proportion of the study population who had experienced such low back pain during the past year was 36%; this is the **one year period prevalence**. The corresponding figure for 'low back pain ever' was 58%; an estimate of the **lifetime prevalence**.

In 1993 the Office of Population Surveys and Censuses (OPCS) carried out an interview-based survey of 6000 adults aged 16 years and above from a random sample of households in Great Britain. The sampling frame for this study was that used in the monthly OPCS Omnibus Surveys, namely the register of postcode addresses of private households. The definition of low back pain was identical to that used in the MRC study, and the one year period prevalence of the symptom was 37%[4].

So these two separate surveys, one based on a self-completion questionnaire and one on an interview, produced very similar prevalence figures. This underlines the value of symptom reporting if identical, explicit case definitions are employed. The OPCS survey did not ask about back pain ever, but did enquire about low back pain on the day of interview. This **point** prevalence was 14%.

A third British survey, of an adult population sample in South Manchester, used the same questions and pain mannikin also[5]. This study addressed the question of whether non-response in population surveys results in a biased estimate of back pain prevalence. Do non-responders for example fail to complete a questionnaire because none of them have back pain? The Manchester study compared prevalence in those who responded immediately and those who delayed until a first or second reminder; it also compared subsequent consultation rates for low back pain in general practice between survey responders and non-responders. The conclusion was that bias is likely to be small. Survey responders provide a good picture of self-reported back pain in the community.

The lone observation that low back pain is common would not justify such elaborate prevalence surveys. A crucial aspect of such studies is to estimate the extent to which low back pain has a significant impact on people's lives.

4. How disabling is low back pain?

The impact of low back pain can be measured by general scales of functional health (such as the Nottingham Health Profile) or by back pain-specific schedules. Several of the latter type are in use, including questionnaires used in the two recent UK surveys, an instrument developed in British primary care by Roland and Morris[6] and a more recent scheme developed in Aberdeen and based on the short-form 36 general instrument[7] (see Chapter 2).

One useful measure of disability is 'Total time in the past year during which back pain sufferers have experienced their pain', an idea developed by American researchers[8]. In the OPCS survey 12% of adults in the general British population had experienced more than 3 months of low back pain in the twelve months prior to the survey[4]. In any one month, one in 10 people in the OPCS study had had to restrict their activity because of low back pain, whilst 7% had not worked because of low back pain. Walsh and colleagues employed a scoring scheme based on the number and severity of reported restrictions of daily living, on a scale from 0 to 16[5]. During a twelve month period approximately 6% of their adult population had a score of 9 or more. These figures suggest that about 1 in 4 adults with low back pain during the course of one year will experience significant impact on their daily living activity as a result. This contrasts with the figure of 80% of low back sufferers in the OPCS survey whose back pain problems had initially started prior to the year in question: intermittent and episodic problems are the rule, and chronicity alone is a poor discriminator of severity.

5. Health care utilisation

In Britain the gatekeeper function of primary care provides a unique epidemiological opportunity. Morbidity data from general practitioners provides a good estimate of the incidence of the problem in the population as reflected in care seeking behaviour, *i.e.* consultation with the family doctor. It will not necessarily include Accident and Emergency attendances, and it will exclude consultations with practitioners outside the health care system. However the OPCS study indicated that the number of people with low back pain in Britain who visit complementary practitioners is small compared with the volume of back pain consultations in general practice.

The main sources of data on consultations for low back pain are the National Morbidity Surveys in General Practice, conducted by the Royal College of General Practitioners in collaboration with the Department of Health and OPCS. There have been four such surveys since 1955, an approximate ten year cycle. Each survey lasts for one year, and is based on a group of volunteer practices, who collect and record data on all contacts with patients during the study period.

The Fourth Morbidity Survey was completed in 1992[9]. Out of every 10,000 patients registered with a general practitioner, 750 (7.5%) consulted at least once in the course of the study year with a back problem considered to be musculoskeletal in origin. The consultation rate was 1350 consultations per 10,000 registered population, suggesting an average of about 2 consultations per patient with a back problem per year. The majority of patients who consulted in the course of a year were considered by the recording GP to have a new episode of the back problem. In the South Manchester cohort study, in which a population sample of adults was followed up for one year to identify those who consulted their general practitioner with low back pain, most consulters had experienced back trouble before, suggesting that consultations are usually about recurrence or exacerbation rather than a 'first ever' episode.

An important point for interpretation of the RCGP survey is that such figures represent both the patients' decision to consult and the doctors' perception of the nature of the main presenting problem. Diagnostic criteria are not formulated in advance in such studies, so that the best interpretation is that they represent "the incidence of consultation for all conditions regarded by the GP as concerned primarily with the low back". In this context it is hardly surprising that the most frequent category assigned to back patients by the general practitioners was 'unspecified disorders of the back' (372 per 100,000 registered patients) followed by sprains and strains of the back (212 per 100,000).

The second point is that the study participants were not representative of all GPs - the volunteer practices were likely to under-represent working populations, particularly inner city groups. That this might be important was one intriguing finding reported by Walsh's team[3]. They showed that there was a four-fold increased propensity to consult for low back pain in the study area with the highest consultation rate (Peterlee, a new town in the North of England) compared with the lowest (St. Austell in Cornwall). This could not be explained by an equivalent variation in the prevalence of low back pain in the respective populations. It is likely that such differences relate primarily to variations in consulting behaviour from practice to practice rather than that the RCGP figures are unrepresentative of the country as a whole.

From such figures it can be estimated that at any one time fewer than one-fifth of all those who have low back pain consult because of it.

During one year 10-20% of low back sufferers seen in primary care are referred to a hospital specialist, and 15-20% are referred for a lumbar spine X-ray. These figures vary widely between practices. Waddell has summarised available data on the proportion of the adult population seen by physical therapists for low back pain each year in Britain: 3.6% by physiotherapists, 1.5% by osteopaths, 0.6% by chiropractors[10]. Again regional variations are likely to be large.

6. The clinical epidemiology of low back pain

Diagnosis is an important issue in assessing the individual patient with low back pain. However there is a general acceptance that most cases of low back pain are 'non-specific'. One contribution that epidemiology can make to the diagnostic process is to supply background data about the relationship between low back pain and specific spinal diagnoses.

Take, for example, the radiographic reporting of 'degenerative disc disease' in the spine. There is no specific definition of this which is generally accepted. In their 1958 paper on radiographic osteoarthrosis and disc degeneration in the general population, Kellgren and Lawrence took the latter to include osteophytosis of the vertebral bodies and narrowing of the disc space[2]. In their unique random sample of spinal radiographs from a survey of adults in a Lancashire town, the prevalence of moderate-to-severe lumbar disc degeneration was 18%, higher in males than females. Minor changes were much commoner (a further 37% affected). However a history of low back pain obtained on the day that the X-rays were taken was no more likely to be positive among those who were subsequently found to have degenerative disc disease in the lumbar spine than among those with no such changes.

The finding that there is no overall relationship between spinal disc disease on X-ray and low back pain has been confirmed in studies using more advanced imaging techniques. Subsequent work, for example using magnetic resonance imaging (by British groups among others), has revealed how common disc abnormalities are in the general population, and that they are only a little more likely to be found in those with low back pain compared with those who are free of the symptom[11]. The importance of detailed imaging of the spine to aid diagnosis in the individual back sufferer has been well outlined elsewhere in this book (Chapters 5-7); but as a means to characterise the symptom epidemiologically, it is flawed because low back pain is not equivalent to spinal disease in the general population.

Given the uncertainties of diagnostic categorisation, the clinical epidemiology of non-specific back pain has focused on characteristics which may predict outcome. Studies of general practice consulters (*e.g.* that of Roland and colleagues[12]) have emphasised that a recent history of back pain and a long symptom duration at first presentation are associated with poorer outcomes 12 months later. Physical signs (other than straight leg raising in the Roland study) have not proved to be particularly helpful in predicting outcome. There is now a strong strand of British studies, from workers such as Klenerman[13] and Main[14], who have demonstrated clearly that psychological factors are the strongest predictors of outcome in hospital, accident and emergency, and general practice patients presenting with low back pain.

7. Risk factors for low back pain

7.1. Age

Although complaints of low back pain do appear to rise with age in the general population, the British surveys[3-5] indicate that this is not a sharp rise. First the cumulative prevalence of low back pain is already 40% by the age of 30 years. Second there is a decline in the prevalence of current low back pain in the elderly. The reasons for the latter are unclear; the possibilities are:

(a) a true decline in episode incidence in the elderly, because of the absence of occupational triggers for example,
(b) higher reporting thresholds in the elderly,
(c) less back pain in those who are generally healthier and who 'survive' to older ages,
(d) a cohort effect (meaning that the current generation of older people might have been less prone to low back pain throughout their lives).

7.2. Gender

Like age, gender differences are considerably less marked for low back pain than they are for other musculoskeletal problems[3-5]. Consultations for back pain are rather higher among women than men, but no higher than expected from the generally higher levels of consultation.

Hormonal factors have been raised as important influences on low back pain. A recent British study confirmed that parity is associated with reported low back pain: the more children a woman has had, the more likely they are to report low back pain[15]. However, a hormonal explanation for this was questioned because the same study found a similar association in men, raising the possibility of a biomechanical or socio-economic reason for the link. Another British study - a prospective study of women followed after childbirth - has identified one possible risk factor in parous women, namely the use of epidural anaesthesia[16]. In this study MacArthur and colleagues followed up 11,701 women after childbirth, and found an episode incidence of low back pain of 18% in women who had had an epidural compared with 10% in those who had not.

A major contribution to the epidemiology of common symptoms in women in Britain has been the cohort study of the health effects of the oral contraceptive pill of the Royal College of General Practitioners. There was no clear link between consultations for low back pain in that cohort and current or previous use of the pill[17].

7.3. Socioeconomic factors

In cross-sectional population studies there is a consistent link between social and economic factors and low back pain. In men, manual occupational class is associated with a higher reported level of low back pain. This might result from the effects of heavy or awkward physical loading at work, but the same relationship in women, for example, appeared more strongly associated with low household income than with occupational class as such[18].

There is a strong inverse trend of rising general practice consultation rates for low back pain across social class categories in both men and women: the lower the social class, the higher the consultation rate[9]. This was not explained by any general association between consultation rates for all conditions and social class.

One problem with cross-sectional population surveys which examine such relationships is that they cannot disentangle cause and effect and they tend to identify proportionately more chronic problems - so it may be that the socioeconomic link is one with chronicity or disability rather than with low back pain *per se*. However prospective data is accumulating to support the notion that socioeconomic factors can influence the incidence of new episodes of low back pain.

7.4. Psychological factors

Closely allied to the socioeconomic issue is the influence of psychological factors. Pioneering occupational cohort studies by Troup and others indicated that biomechanical factors alone did not explain the variance observed in the rate of occurrence of new low back pain episodes in the workforce[19]. In the South Manchester cohort, 1638 adult subjects identified in a population sample as being free of current low back pain were followed up for one year[20]. The likelihood of a new episode of low back pain starting during the year was directly related to baseline levels of depression, anxiety, job satisfaction and perceived income levels at baseline, confirming earlier observations from occupational cohorts here and in America. More recently the Huddersfield group have shown a reduction in the incidence of new episodes of low back pain among factory workers given a simple leaflet which addressed perceptions and cognitions around low back pain[21].

7.5. Physical and anthropometric factors

Height and weight have been a focus of interest as possible causes of low back pain. Intuitively, loading of the spine would be expected to cause low back pain. In the Health Survey there was an association between body mass index (BMI) and low back pain, with a clear trend in women of rising prevalence of low back pain with increasing BMI[18]. The surveys of Kellgren and Lawrence suggested that X-ray changes in the spine were more common in obese men than in non-obese men[2]. In the MRC studies there was a doubling of the likelihood of reporting low back pain among men in the tallest quintile compared with those in the shortest, a relationship not explained by selection into different occupations according to height[22].

7.6. Other lifestyle factors

Smoking is important for two reasons. Its consistent association with low back pain in cross-sectional population studies[18] suggests that the reduction in smoking prevalence could have an important influence on low back pain occurrence. Secondly there are plausible explanations for the association, namely chronic coughing and poor nutrition of the intervertebral disc.

Occupational activity is an important risk, reviewed elsewhere, but in the general population the more important question concerns the general influence of physical activity. Here, cross-sectional studies may be crucially misleading since the effect of low back pain on physical activity levels is likely to be marked. This has yet to be investigated in the British setting, although studies from abroad are beginning to indicate that general physical activity is good for the back.

7.7. General physical health

Linked to this is the general issue of the concurrence of problems in patients with low back pain. Given such a common symptom, it is not surprising that patients report other problems - but this happens more frequently than can be explained by chance. Cross-sectional studies in the general population indicate that concurrence of pain syndromes is common, whilst prospective studies have recently shown that general physical poor health is a strong predictor of new episodes of low back pain[20].

Walsh and colleagues, in their population-based study, examined the risk of low back pain in relation to a previous admission to hospital because of a traffic accident or fall. They concluded that such an event conferred a 7% additional risk of developing low back pain subsequently[23].

Studies in primary care and in the general population confirm that the strongest predictor of new episodes of low back pain is a history of previous such episodes.

8. Prevention

The ultimate justification of epidemiological studies of the causes of low back pain in the British population is that they will lead to effective means to prevent the problem.

Waddell's excellent account of the phenomenal rise, during the past two decades, in work loss and invalidity payments arising from low back pain makes it clear that this 'epidemic' is about more than just a medical condition[10]. It is about economic and employment factors, the nature of the welfare state, the opportunity for rehabilitation, and the extent to which low back pain is in fact a general problem of work disability and invalidity rather than a specific medical condition. Waddell argues that the 'epidemic' of low back pain is essentially an epidemic of work disability and has to be tackled as such.

Such a view does not rule out more general preventive approaches. The ideal is primary prevention - to prevent the problem occurring in the first place - but since the experience of low back pain is so common by early adulthood, it is more realistic to think in terms of secondary prevention - reducing the frequency and persistence of low back episodes. The extent to which the latter can be attributed to poor general physical fitness, smoking, and being overweight, holds out the hope that general health improvements - important for the prevention of other problems, musculoskeletal and otherwise - will help to reduce the burden of low back pain.

Although the social and psychological roots of low back pain persistence might appear to be firmly entrenched in our society, here again the notion of secondary prevention holds out hope. The extent to which the mechanism of pain persistence rests on inappropriate attitudes and beliefs about low back pain holds out the possibility of large scale influence through methods such as that studied by Main[14] and the Huddersfield group[31] - simple education directed at altering attitudes and beliefs. Coupled with appropriate treatment of depression and anxiety states, psychological approaches to prevention could have a considerable impact, even though root causes of unhappiness and job dissatisfaction persist.

Finally the ergonomic and rehabilitation approaches provide preventive potential in specific occupational settings, allied to legislation on manual handling for example which represents the 'primary preventive' approach in industry. The health service has its own problems here: Smedley and colleagues, among others, have reported the high prevalence of low back pain in nurses[24]. The impact which workplace interventions have on low back pain as a whole will depend not only on their effective implementation, but also on the contribution which occupation makes to the total occurrence of low back pain in the general population.

9. References

1. B.D. Cox, Health and lifestyle survey 1984-5 (computer file). ESRC data archive. Colchester, 1988.

2. J.S. Lawrence, *Ann. Rheum. Dis.* **28** (1969) 121.

3. K. Walsh, M. Cruddas and D. Coggon, *J. Epidemiol. Community Health* **46** (1992) 227.

4. V. Mason, The prevalence of back pain in Great Britain, Office of Population Censuses and Surveys, Social Survey Division. (HMSO, London, 1994).

5. A. Papageorgiou, P.R. Croft, S. Ferry, M.I.V. Jayson and A. Silman, *Spine* **20** (1995) 1889.

6. M. Roland and R. Morris, *Spine* **8** (1983) 141.

7. D.A. Ruta, A.M. Garratt, D. Wardlaw and I.T. Russell, *Spine* **19** (1994) 1887.

8. M. von Korff, J. Ormel, F. Keefe and S.F. Dworkin, *Pain* **50** (1992) 133.

9. A. McCormick, D. Fleming, J. Charlton, Morbidity statistics from general practice. Fourth national study 1991-1992, Office of Population Censuses and Surveys, Series MB5 no. 3. (HMSO, London, 1995).

10. Clinical Standards Advisory Group on Back Pain. Back pain : epidemiology and costs. (HMSO, London, 1994).

11. M.C. Powell, M. Wilson, P. Szypryt, E.M. Symonds and B.S. Worthington, *Lancet* **2** (1986) 1366.

12. M.O. Roland, D.C. Morrell and R.W. Morris, *Brit. Med. J.* **286** (1983) 523.

13. L. Klenerman, P.D. Slade, I.M. Stanley, B. Pennie, J.P. Reilly, L.E. Atchison, J.D.G. Troup and M.J. Rose, *Spine* **20** (1995) 478.

14. C.J. Main, P.L.R. Wood, S. Hollis, C.C. Spanswick and G. Waddell, *Spine* **17** (1991) 42.

15.   A.J. Silman, S. Ferry, A.C. Papageorgiou, M.I.V. Jayson and P.R. Croft, *Arthr. Rheum.* **38** (1995) 1232.

16.   C. MacArthur, M. Lewis, E.G. Knox and J.S. Crawford, *Brit. Med. J.* **301** (1990) 9.

17.   P. Hannaford, Personal communication, Royal College of General Practitioners Manchester Research Unit.

18.   P.R. Croft and, A.S. Rigby, *J. Epidemiol. Community Health* **48** (1994) 166.

19.   J.D.G. Troup and T. Videman, *Clin. Biomech.* **4** (1989) 173.

20.   P.R. Croft, A.C. Papageorgiou, S. Ferry, E. Thomas, M.I.V. Jayson and A.J. Silman, *Spine* **20** (1995) 2731.

21.   T.L. Symonds, A.K. Burton, K.M. Tillotson and C.J. Main, *Spine* **20** (1995) 2738.

22.   K. Walsh, M. Cruddas and D. Coggon, *Scand. J. Work Env. Health* **17** (1991) 420.

23.   K. Walsh, M. Cruddas and D. Coggon, *J. Epidemiol. Community Health* **46** (1992) 231.

24.   J. Smedley, P. Egger, C. Cooper and D. Coggon, *Occupational and Environmental Medicine* **52** (1995) 160.

CHAPTER 2

MEASURING HEALTH OUTCOMES IN LOW BACK PAIN

A. Garratt and D. Ruta

1. Introduction

There are a number of different approaches to measuring patient perceptions of health outcomes for patients suffering from low back pain. First we shall provide a framework for the different approaches to measuring outcomes and consider the necessary criteria for a valid measure. Then, the instruments that have been used for assessing the outcomes of patients with low back pain are considered in the light of these criteria.

2. Measuring patient perceptions of health outcomes

Traditional measures of physiological, physical or psychological impairment have long used by clinicians to assess the effects of medical care on their patients. In recent years, however, the appropriateness of these clinical indicators as measures of 'health' outcome has been called into question[17,31,44]. Although their appeal lies in their objectivity and availability through routine collection, they appear to lack the ability to predict clinically relevant outcomes such as functional capacity[17]. Perhaps more importantly, such measurements do not necessarily reflect the way the patient feels or functions. If the goal of medical care is to improve the quality of life of patients then outcomes measurement should be directed towards assessing improvements in quality of life which are a direct consequence of medical care, such as functional status and well-being.

2.1. Specific and generic measures of health outcome

Broadly speaking, there are two approaches to measuring patient perceptions about the outcomes of health care: specific instruments that focus on a particular disease or client group, and generic instruments that provide a summary of overall health. Both approaches have their strengths and weaknesses and, for the purposes of measuring health outcomes, there are potential advantages to using the two in conjunction[53]. In theory, the narrow focus of specific instruments may make them more responsive or sensitive to clinically important changes in health resulting from health care interventions[37,53,26]. Specific instruments can be selected that reflect the areas considered by patients or clinicians to be of greatest importance and can be specific to a particular disease, population, function, condition, or problem. Generic instruments can take account of multiple conditions enabling them to measure wider effects such as the influence of co-morbidity on health. Their general nature makes them suitable for comparisons between different groups of patients and general or disease-free populations[42,15]. Generic instruments have greater potential to capture unforeseen effects and side effects of an intervention which may go undetected by a specific instrument. This makes them potentially useful for assessing the impact of new health care technologies when the therapeutic effects are uncertain.

There are two major classes of generic instrument: health profiles and utility measures. Health profiles measure health across a number of distinct areas or dimensions including, for example, physical functioning, mental health and role limitations. The items within health profiles are scored and summed to reflect the individual dimensions and sometimes produce a single score or overall summary of health. Examples of health profiles include the Sickness Impact Profile[2], the Nottingham Health Profile[23] and the Short Form 36-Item Health Survey (SF-36)[51]. The broad focus of health profiles enables comparisons to be made across different conditions which is useful for economic evaluation, including cost-effectiveness analysis, where outcomes are expressed in natural units - *eg.* cost per percentage improvement in physical function. Health profiles are not, however, suitable for cost-utility analysis which takes account of the preferences or values associated with health related quality of life (HRQL) states. Utility measures incorporate the values attached to individual health states and express HRQL states as a single index. Through the process of valuing health states and the duration of those states Quality Adjusted Life Years (QALYs) are produced[55]. QALY valuations can be calculated either by eliciting values directly from patients or by using a third party such as the general public. The Euroqol instrument asks subjects to complete five items covering mobility, self-care, main activity, pain/discomfort and anxiety/depression[11]. Combinations of possible responses, or HRQL states, have been valued by third parties so that states are expressed as utility values between 0 (worst possible state) and 1 (best possible state). On the basis of their responses to the five Euroqol items patients are classified into a HRQL state which has a utility value associated with it.

2.2. Assessing measures of health outcome

To be of practical value a measure of outcome must satisfy the criteria of validity, reliability, responsiveness and practicality. Validity refers to an instrument's ability to measure what is intended. In the absence of a 'gold standard' measure of HRQL, validity is usually assessed through construct validity, or how an instrument should behave in relation to some theory or construct. Reliability refers to an instrument's ability to measure something in a consistent manner and can be assessed through internal consistency, which assesses the level of agreement between questions that measure related aspects of health, and test-retest, which assesses the stability of an instrument over repeated administrations. For instruments designed to measure outcome, it has been argued that test-retest is the most appropriate method of assessing reliability[29]. Responsiveness refers to the ability of an instrument to detect clinically important changes in health. Several methods have been suggested for assessing responsiveness. Typically, the change scores of instruments are compared after the introduction of some intervention of known efficacy[26,27]. Finally, instruments must be practical, that is they should be easy to administer and be acceptable to patients. The issue of practicality is related to the application of the instrument. For example, an instrument that is being used in routine clinical practice for audit purposes will have to satisfy more stringent requirements in terms of administrative costs than an instrument being used as part of a clinical trial.

2.3. Reliability

The standard for assessing test-retest reliability is the intraclass correlation coefficient[10], but Pearson's correlation coefficient is more readily available on computer packages. Pearson's correlation coefficient does not take account of systematic bias and can overestimate reliability[43]. This statistic has been supplemented with analysis of the distributions of score differences which indicates if there is any systematic bias[40].

2.4. Validity

In the absence of a "gold standard" measure of HRQL validity is usually assessed by recourse to clinical or social theory. Instruments have been assessed for validity through comparisons with other instruments that measure related phenomena[25,39] and by relating their scores to clinical and laboratory data and sociodemographic variables[14].

2.5. Responsiveness

Whilst there exist generally agreed methods for assessing the validity and reliability of HRQL instruments[44] there is no standard technique for assessing the responsiveness or sensitivity of instruments to clinical change[10,46]. Several methods for assessing responsiveness are available but the relative merits of these approaches are not yet fully understood. The methods can be grouped according to: first, the context in which the instrument is applied, for example, researchers have assessed responsiveness following interventions or by following up patients after some time interval; and secondly the different methods used to quantify responsiveness, for example, effect sizes which relate changes in scores derived from instruments to the standard deviation of the scores.

Previous work has related change scores on measures of health outcome to external criteria and processes of care. The degree of concordance between change scores on HRQL instruments and external criteria has been assessed using transition questions and clinical data. Transition questions ask the patient or clinician to judge whether there has been a change in health[4,7,32]. In a similar way change scores have been related to clinical and laboratory measures[24] - *eg.* clinicians' assessment of severity. In relating outcomes to processes of care, several studies have looked at changes in the scores on instruments following interventions of known efficacy including total joint arthroplasty[30] and total hip arthroplasty[27].

Several methods have been proposed for quantifying the responsiveness of outcome measures. These include mean differences and significance levels[21], receiver operator characteristic curves[8,32], Guyatt's index of responsiveness[20], effect sizes[28] and standardised response means[30]. Through comparisons of the significance levels of HRQL changes the responsiveness of different instruments can be compared[21]. Receiver operator characteristic (ROC) curves assess the predictive ability of instruments in relation to some external criterion of change[8]. Using this method to assess responsiveness is similar to assessing a diagnostic test. As with a diagnostic test a change in the score generated by an instrument can be described in terms of its sensitivity and specificity using the external criterion of change. ROC curve analysis does allow statistical comparisons across instruments but requires a dichotomous external criterion which limits the extent to which instruments can be assessed and compared in terms of their responsiveness and in particularly the magnitude of responsiveness.

The methods that follow are not dependent upon a dichotomous criterion for assessing change and as such are capable of providing information about the magnitude of responsiveness. The first is known as effect size which equals the mean change in scores divided by the baseline standard deviation of the scores[13,28]. A variant of this approach is Guyatt's index of responsiveness[20] which has the same numerator but the denominator is equal to the standard deviation of score changes among stable subjects. Setting the numerator equal to the smallest score difference that is clinically significant gives direct estimates of the sample sizes required in clinical trials. However, a problem with this approach is the method of estimating score changes for the stable subjects to use in the denominator. Estimates could be derived using the test-retest method of assessing reliability, however, there are problems with this approach, in particular subjects may have really changed between the two intervals of administration which would result in an underestimate of responsiveness. The standardised response mean (SRM)[27,30], which is equal to the mean change in scores divided by the standard deviation of the score differences, is another form of effect size statistic. The SRM has an important advantage over the other methods in that it is a standardised measure that enables comparisons to be made between different instruments using statistical testing[30].

2.6. Practicality

Practical considerations, including the length and mode of administration should also be taken into account when assessing the suitability of outcome measures. If multiple measures of outcome are being used, for example generic and specific instruments, then questionnaire length is an important consideration. Instruments that have a long completion time are less suitable when time is an important factor, for example in a clinical setting where instruments are being routinely administered. Instruments that require administration by interview are less practical. For example, if patients are being followed up with a questionnaire following hospital treatment interview administration would be more costly than postal or telephone administration of the questionnaire.

3. Outcome measures for patients with low back pain

The previous section highlights the importance of using specific and generic instruments in conjunction so that all treatment effects are captured. Both types of instrument have been used in the patient assessment of outcomes for low back pain. This section looks at the relative merits of the generic and specific instruments that have been used in relation to the criteria of validity, reliability, responsiveness and practicality.

3.1. Generic instruments

Two of the most widely used generic instruments in patients with low back pain are the Sickness Impact Profile (SIP)[2] and the Short-Form 36-Item Health Survey Questionnaire (SF-36)[52]. The SIP and the SF-36 are measures of HRQL that are designed to be applicable to a broad range of illnesses of varying severity and can be used for measuring the outcomes of care. The SIP consists of 136 items that ask about health-related dysfunction in 12 areas of activity. It can be self- or interview-administered and takes an average of 25 minutes to complete. An overall SIP score and scores for each of the 12 areas of activity can be generated as a percentage. The instrument has been used across a wide range of illnesses including low back pain[8]. The SF-36 is a more recent addition to the HRQL literature but is in wide use. The instrument comprises 36 items that measure three aspects of health: functional status, well-being, and overall evaluation of health using eight separate scales. The responses to the items on each scale are summed to produce eight scores between 0 (worst possible) and 100 (best possible).

The reliability coefficients of both instruments have been found to satisfy accepted standards in a variety of patient groups[2,40]. A test-retest reliability coefficient of 0.85 has been demonstrated for the overall SIP score in a low back pain patient group[6]. For the eight SF-36 scales test-retest reliability coefficients ranging from 0.66 to 0.93 were found in four patient groups which included patients with low back pain[40]. For the low back pain subgroup reliability coefficients range from 0.65 to 0.90 (Garratt, unpublished data). Similarly, there is a large amount of published evidence supporting the validity of the two instruments as measures of HRQL across a variety of illnesses. The validity of the two instruments in patients with low back pain has been assessed by the same authors[6,15,39]. Moderate correlations were found between the SIP and various biological and clinical measures[6]. In another study of patients with low back pain moderate correlations were found between the subscales of the SIP and the Minnesota Multiphasic Personality Inventory[14]. Evidence for the validity of the SF-36 in low back pain patients was demonstrated by the statistically significant association with a series of hypothetical constructs. Scores derived from the eight scales of the SF-36 were related to general practitioners ratings of symptom severity; related to use and strength of analgesics; and were higher in referred than non-referred patients[15,39]. The scores of the low back pain patients were also found to deviate from those of the general population in a way that had clinical validity[15].

The responsiveness of the SIP and SF-36 has also been assessed in a variety of illnesses[7,16,27,30,32] including low back pain[8,14,16,39]. Deyo and Centor used t-statistics and ROC curves to assess the responsiveness of the SIP using a global assessment of improvement as an external criterion. In patients who had improved significant changes in SIP scores and subscales were found and the ROC curve analysis showed that the SIP was able to discriminate between improved and unimproved patients[8]. In assessing the responsiveness of the SF-36, Garratt and co-workers found a significant relationship between changes on the SF-36 scales and self reported health transition in four patient groups including low back pain. Across all eight SF-36 scales significant improvements were found for patients managed within general practice and those referred to specialists with their back pain[16]. In back pain patients reporting a change in their general health over a two week period standardised response means representing a small to moderate change were found for six of the eight scales of the SF-36[39]. A comparison of the responsiveness of the SIP and SF-36 was made for patients undergoing total hip arthroplasty[27]. The largest SRMs were found for three of the SF-36 scales which represented a large effect.

The practicality of the two instruments is dependent on their length, mode of administration and ease of completion. Both instruments can be self-completed which is an important consideration if patients are to be followed up outwith the clinical setting. The SF-36 is the more practical of the two instruments taking only 10 minutes to complete compared to the SIP which takes 25 minutes to complete. Short-form instruments such as the SF-36 have been developed in response to the need for practical instruments that can be quickly administered routinely in clinical settings. The lengthy completion time of the SIP was an important consideration in the development of a specific instrument for back pain patients which draws on SIP items for content[38].

3.2. Specific instruments

Two reviews of specific measures of outcome for low back pain have recently been undertaken[3,39]. Both assessed the instruments in relation to the criteria of validity, reliability and responsiveness. Ruta *et al.* compared the Aberdeen Low Back Pain Scale with three other instruments that measure more than just the impairment associated with low back pain: the Low Back Outcome Score, the Waddell Disability Index and the Oswestry Disability Questionnaire[39]. A more recent review compared the four most widely applied measures of functional status intended for assessing the outcomes of patients with low back pain: the Oswestry Disability Questionnaire, the Million Visual Analogue Scale, the Roland Disability Questionnaire and the Waddell Disability Index[3].

The Low Back Outcome Scale[18] and The Million Visual Analogue Scale[36] have been subjected to little or no formal testing for responsiveness to change and despite being published for some time there is relatively less published work on their other properties. The review that follows focuses on four instruments: the Oswestry Disability Questionnaire, the Roland Disability Questionnaire, the Waddell Disability Index and the Aberdeen Low Back Pain Scale. The Oswestry Disability Questionnaire attempts to measure the extent to which daily activities are affected by back pain[12]. No information is available for its conceptual basis. The instrument consists of ten items that cover pain, self-care, lifting, walking, standing, sleeping, sex life, social life and travelling. Responses to the items are summed and rescaled to produce a score between 0 and 100, with higher values representing greater disability. The instrument has undergone modifications[32,33] and similar levels of validity and reliability have been found for the different versions of the instrument[22].

The Roland Disability Questionnaire was derived from items within the Sickness Impact Profile that cover a range of aspects of daily living[38]. The 24 items selected from the SIP represent the areas of greatest relevance to low back pain. To make the instrument specific to back pain the phrase "because of my back pain" was added to each of the items. As in the SIP the items consist of the yes/no response format and scores can vary from 0 (no disability) to 24 (severe disability).

The Waddell Disability Index is designed to measure the affect of low back pain on physical activities of daily living[48]. The instrument consists of nine items derived from previous work[55] and pilot interviews and includes lifting, sitting, standing, walking, sleeping, social activity, sexual life and putting on footwear. The responses to the items are of a yes/no format and are summed to produce a score out of nine with higher values representing greater levels of disability.

In the development of the Aberdeen Back Pain Scale a review of the clinical literature was undertaken and items selected that reflect the areas of importance in the clinical assessment of patients with low back pain[39]. The resulting items were then assessed by a Consultant orthopaedic surgeon specialising in the treatment of low back pain, a rheumatologist and a physiotherapist with a special interest in low back pain. The areas covered include duration of pain, duration of analgesia, effect of lying down, areas of pain, areas of weakness and loss of feeling, bending, sleep, work, confinement to bed, sex life, leisure and self care. The instrument consists of 19 items that are either a forced choice (tick one box) or a multiple choice format (tick all boxes that apply) and are summed and rescaled to produce a "back pain severity score" between 0 and 100.

The tests of reliability of the four instruments are summarised in Table 1. For the instruments that have been assessed for test-retest reliability - the Oswestry Disability Questionnaire, the Roland Disability Questionnaire and the Aberdeen Low Back Pain Scale - the reliability estimates, as measured by the correlation coefficient, are above the level of 0.7 which is acceptable for comparing groups of patients. The reliability of the Oswestry and the Roland instruments has been assessed by several studies and all produced satisfactory estimates. For the purpose of comparison, where possible, studies incorporating the same time interval between test and retest are presented. Also included are the results of studies that have calculated reliability estimates based on the intraclass correlation coefficient. The two reliability estimates for the Aberdeen instrument are based on the same data whereas those for the Oswestry are from separate studies. For the Aberdeen instrument the intraclass and Pearson coefficients are of the same magnitude of 0.94 whereas the intraclass correlation coefficient for the Oswestry instrument is somewhat lower at 0.83. Instruments with reliability estimates as high as 0.94 are suitable for individual as well as group comparisons[43]. In comparing instruments for reliability consideration should be given to the design of the test-retest studies. For example, the Aberdeen Low Back Pain Scale was assessed for test-retest after a two week interval compared to the same day for the other two instruments. Shorter time intervals between test and retest limit the possibility for changes in health which would result in an underestimate of reliability. However, it is possible that patients are more likely to remember their previous responses which can result in an overestimate of reliability.

Table 1. Reliability Testing of the Specific Instruments

	Oswestry Disability Questionnaire	Roland Disability Questionnaire	Waddell Disability Index	Aberdeen Low Back Pain Scale
Pearson's Correlation Coefficient	0.94 (same day)[12]	0.91 (same day)[37]	n/a	0.94 (2 weeks)[38]
Intra-class Correlation Coefficient	0.83 (1 week)[19]			0.94 (2 weeks)[a]

[a]Garratt (unpublished data)

Lumbar Spine Disorders: Current Concepts

Table 2. Validity testing of the specific instruments

	Generic Instruments	Specific Instruments	Clinical
Oswestry Disability Questionnaire		Low Back Outcome[18], Pain Disability Index[19], Roland Disability Questionnaire[48], Waddell Disability Index[48], VAS pain rating[19]. $0.47 < r < 0.87$	Presence/absence of relaxation in back muscles during flexion, trunk mobility/strength distribution of paraspinal muscle atrophy $0.33 < r < 0.74$[45]
Roland Disability Questionnaire	SIP (r =0.85)[8]	Oswestry Disability Questionnaire[5], McGill Pain Questionnaire[25], Pain Disability Index[34], Functional Assessment Screening Questionnaire[34], VAS pain rating[38], self-rated improvement[8], Professional-rated improvement[8], Pain drawing[25], Return to full activity[8]. $0.27 < r < 0.77$	Combined physical tests[51], Spinal flexion[8], Improvements in spinal flexion[8]. $0.29 < r < 0.51$
Waddell Disability Index		Low Back Outcome Scale[18], Oswestry Disability Questionnaire[48]. $0.70 < r < 0.77$	Combination of physical tests[51], Physical Impairment Index[47], Spinal flexion[47]. $0.30 < r < 0.60$
Aberdeen Low Back Pain Scale	SF-36 $(0.36 < r < 0.69)$[39]		GP ratings of symptom severity, Analgesic use, Referred or not[39]. $(P<0.05)$

r = Pearson's correlation coefficient

The tests of validity for the four instruments are summarised in Table 2. The largest amount of evidence, derived from seven studies, is available for the Roland Disability Questionnaire which has been subjected to comparisons with generic instruments, specific instruments and clinical data. It follows that the instrument had a large correlation with the SIP, from which the Roland instrument was derived[8]. The instrument was also found to have significant correlations of a small to moderate magnitude with several other specific instruments, some of which have been subjected to separate tests for validity, including the Oswestry Disability[5] and the McGill Pain Questionnaires[25]. Small to moderate correlations

Table 3. Responsiveness testing of the specific instruments

	Setting	Method of Assessment	Comparison with other instruments
Oswestry Disability Questionnaire	Statistically significant improvement in patients expected to improve 3 weeks post-treatment[12]	t-test	
Roland Disability Questionnaire	Statistically significant improvement in patients judged to have improved[8]	t-test and ROC curve analysis	Similar level of responsiveness as SIP
Waddell Disability Index	Statistically significant improvement in patients judged to be clinically successful[48]	t-test	
Aberdeen Low Back Pain Scale	Statistically significant deterioration in patients with poorer health[39]	Standardised response mean	More responsive than SF-36

were found between the Roland instrument and clinical data including physical tests and spinal flexion[8,51]. The Oswestry Disability Questionnaire and the Waddell Disability Index have not been compared with generic instruments but a large amount of evidence has accumulated from comparisons with other specific instruments and clinical data. The Oswestry was found to have moderate to large correlations with several other specific instruments, some of which have undergone separate tests for validity, including the Low Back Outcome Scale[18], the Roland Disability Questionnaire[48] and the Waddell Disability Index[48]. Small to moderate correlations have been found between the instrument and clinical data, including muscle relaxation during spinal flexion, trunk mobility and trunk strength[45]. The Waddell instrument was found to have moderate correlations with instruments that have been subjected to separate tests for validity - the Low Back Outcome Score and the Oswestry instrument[18,48]. Small to moderate correlations were found between the instrument and clinical data relating to physical impairment, physical tests and spinal flexion[47,51]. The Aberdeen Low Back Pain Scale is the most recent addition to the literature but there is good evidence for its validity in the form of comparisons with the SF-36, an instrument that has been shown to have acceptable levels of validity as a generic measure for patients with low back pain[15]. Correlations between the two instruments were of a small to moderate magnitude for the eight scales of the SF-36 with the largest correlation being with the scale of pain[39]. Finally, the Aberdeen instrument was found to be significantly related to general practitioners assessments of symptom severity, whether the patient was referred or not and analgesic use[39].

The tests of responsiveness for the four instruments are summarised in Table 3. Priority was given to studies which included an accepted method for testing responsiveness and a formal comparison of instruments. A comprehensive review of the responsiveness of the four instruments has been undertaken by Beurskens *et al.*[2]. The Roland Disability Questionnaire and the Aberdeen Low Back Pain Scale have been compared with the SIP and the SF-36 respectively. Similar levels of responsiveness were found for the Roland instrument and the SIP in patients judged to have improved[8]. In patients with self-rated poorer health at two weeks the Aberdeen instrument was found to be more responsive than the eight scales of the SF-36. An SRM indicative of a moderate clinical change was found for the specific instrument compared to SRMs representing a small to moderate clinical change for the SF-36. The Oswestry Disability Index and the Waddell Disability Index have demonstrated responsiveness in trials of known efficacy but have not been formally compared to other instruments[12,39].

All four instruments are fairly brief, taking around five minutes to complete, and have proved acceptable to patients as part of a self-administered format. The short completion times makes each of the instruments a suitable component of a package of measures for assessing the outcomes of care that includes generic as well as specific measures of outcome.

4. Conclusions

To be suitable for use in an evaluative context a measure of health outcome must satisfy the criteria of validity, reliability, responsiveness and practicality. Several instruments are available for assessing patient perceptions of outcomes for low back pain which are both specific and generic in nature. The restricted focus of specific instruments makes them potentially more responsive to the important effects of interventions. Generic instruments provide a summary of health related quality of life and are not fixed to any particular condition or disease making them useful for comparisons across conditions. Their general nature means that they have the potential to capture unforeseen or side effects from interventions. For these reasons it has been recommended that specific and generic instruments are used in conjunction[53].

Evidence for the validity, reliability and responsiveness of two widely used generic instruments - the SIP and the SF-36 - has been found in patients with low back pain. Direct comparisons of the two instruments have shown that the SF-36 is as responsive as the SIP[27]. Taking only ten minutes to complete, compared to 25 minutes for the SIP, the SF-36 is the more practical of the two instruments. The most widely tested specific instruments for low back pain that have been used for assessing outcomes include the Oswestry Disability Questionnaire, the Roland Disability Questionnaire, the Waddell Disability Index and the Aberdeen Low Back Pain Scale. With the exception of the Waddell instrument there is strong evidence for the reliability of the instruments with the Aberdeen instrument having the highest level which make it potentially suitable for use in individual patients. There is good evidence for the validity of all four instruments with the Roland instrument being the most widely applied. Both the Roland and the Aberdeen instruments have been subjected to formal tests of responsiveness and compared to well validated generic instruments. The Roland was found to have similar levels of responsiveness as the SIP and the Aberdeen instrument was more responsive than the SF-36.

Finally, worthy of mention is a relatively new approach to measuring patient perceptions of outcomes which asks individual patients about the areas of their lives that are affected by the condition or disease under consideration[36,41]. The Patient Generated Index (PGI), developed by Ruta *et al.* is a measure of individualised quality of life that asks the patient to list the areas of their life affected by their condition and rate them on a scale and weight them in terms of their relative importance[41]. The PGI aims to quantify the impact of a particular condition in those areas of the patients life in which they would most value an improvement. Evidence for the validity and reliability of the PGI was found for patients with low back pain[41]. Measures of individualised quality of life are still at an early stage in their development but represent an exciting and new approach to the measurement of patient perceptions of health outcomes.

In conclusion, any attempt to measure the impact of health care should incorporate patients' subjective accounts of health outcomes. Specific and generic instruments are complementary and should be used together as part of a package in the overall assessment of patient outcomes. Through the inclusion of multiple measures of outcome in research designs comparisons can be made between instruments, be they generic or specific, that will increase our understanding of their relative merits including responsiveness to clinically important effects.

5. References

1. H. Alantara, K. Tallroth, A. Soukka and M. Heliovaara. *J. Spinal Disorders* **6** (1993) 137.
2. M. Bergner, R.A. Bobbitt, W.B. Carter and B.S. Gilson. *Med. Care* **19** (1981) 787.
3. A.J. Beurskens, H.C. de Vet, A.J. Koke, G.J. van der Heijden and P. G. Knipschild. *Spine* **20** (1995) 1017.
4. A.B. Bindman, D. Keane, N. Lurie, *Med. Care* **28** (1990) 1142.
5. Y.Y. Co, S. Easton and M.W. Maxwell, *J. Manipulative Physiol. Ther.* **16** (1993) 14.
6. R.A. Deyo and A.K. Diehl. *Spine* **8** (1983) 635.
7. R.A. Deyo and T.S. Inui. *Health Services Research* **19** (1984) 275.
8. R.A. Deyo and R.M. Centor, *J. Chron. Dis.* **39** (1986) 897.
9. R.A. Deyo, *Spine* **11** (1986) 951.
10. R.A. Deyo, P. Diehr and D.L. Patrick, *Controlled Clinical Trials* **12** (1991) 142S.
11. Euroqol Group, *Health Policy* **16** (1990) 199.
12. J.C.T. Fairbank, J. Couper, J.B. Davies and J.P. O'Brien, *Physiotherapy* **66** (1980) 271.
13. R. Fitzpatrick, S. Ziebland, C. Jenkinson, A. Mowat and A. Mowat. *Quality in Health Care* **1** (1992) 89.
14. M.J. Follick, T.W. Smith and D.K. Ahern, *Pain* **21** (1985) 67.
15. A.M. Garratt, D.A. Ruta, M.I. Abdalla, K.J. Buckingham and I.T. Russell. *Brit. Med. J.* **306** (1993) 1440.

16.   A.M. Garratt, D.A. Ruta, M.I. Abdalla and I.T. Russell. *Quality in Health Care* **3** (1994) 186.

17.   J.W. Garrett and D.A. Drossman, *Gastroenterology* **99** (1990) 90.

18.   C.G. Greenough and R.D. Fraser, *Spine* **17** (1992) 36.

19.   M. Gronblad, M. Hupli, O. Wennerstrand, *et al.*, *Clinical Journal of Pain* **9** (1993) 189.

20.   G. Guyatt, S. Walter and G. Norman, *J. Chron. Dis.* **2** (1987) 171.

21.   G. Guyatt, A. Mitchell, E.J. Irvine, J. Singer, N. Williams, R. Goodacre and C. Tompkins. *Gastroenterology* **96** (1989) 804.

22.   N. Hudson-Cook, K. Tomes-Nicholson and A. Breen, in *Back Pain: New Approaches to Rehabilitation and Education*, ed. O.M. Roland and J.R. Jenner (Manchester University Press, Manchester, 1989).

23.   S.M. Hunt, J. McEwen and S.P. McKenna, *J. Roy. Coll. General Practitioners* **35** (1985) 185.

24.   C. Jenkinson, S. Ziebland, R. Fitzpatrick, A. Mowat and A. Mowat. *Int. J. Health Sciences* **2** (1991) 189.

25.   M.P. Jensen, S.E. Strom, J. Turner and J.M. Romano, *Pain* **50** (1992) 157.

26.   M.E. Kantz, W.J. Harris, K. Levitsky, J.E. Ware, A.R. Davies, *Med. Care.* **30** (1992) MS240.

27.   J.N. Katz, M.G. Larson, C.B. Phillips, A.H. Fossel and M.H. Liang, *Med. Care* **30** (1992) 917.

28.   L.E. Kazis, J.J. Anderson and R.F. Meenan. *Med. Care* **27** (1989) S178.

29.   B. Kirshner and G.H. Guyatt, *J. Chron Dis* **1** (1985) 27.

30.   M.H. Liang, A.H. Fossel and M.G. Larson, *Med. Care* **28** (1990) 632.

31.   L.D. MacKeigan and D.S. Pathal, *Am. J. Hosp. Pharm.* **49** (1992) 2236.

32.   C.R. MacKenzie, M.E. Charlson, D. DiGioia and K. Kelley, *J. Chron. Dis.* **39** (1986) 429.

33.   T.W. Meade, W. Browne and S. Mellows, *J. Epidemiol. Community Health* **40** (1986) 12.

34.   R.W. Millard and R.H. Jones, *Spine* **16** (1991) 835.

35.   R. Million, W. Hall, K.H. Nilsen, R.D Baker and M.I. Jayson, *Spine* **7** (1992) 204.

36.   C.A. O'Boyle, H. McGhee, A. Hickey, K. O'Malley and C.R.B. Joyce, *Lancet* **339** (1992) 1088.

37.   D.L. Patrick and R.A Deyo, *Med. Care* **27** (1989) S217.

38.   M. Roland and R. Morris, *Spine* **8** (1983) 141.

39.   D.A. Ruta, A.M. Garratt, D. Wardlaw and I.T. Russell, *Spine* **17** (1994) 1887.

40.   D.A. Ruta, M.I. Abdalla, A.M. Garratt, A. Coutts and I.T. Russell. *Quality in Health Care* **3** (1994) 180.

41.   D.A. Ruta, A.M. Garratt, M. Leng, I.T.Russell and L.M. MacDonald. *Med. Care* **32** (1994) 1109.

42.   A.L. Stewart, S. Greenfield, R.D. Hays, K. Wells, M.H. Rogers, S.D. Berry and E.A. McGlynn, *JAMA* **262** (1989) 907.

43.   G.L. Streiner and R.D. Norman. *Health measurement scales: A practical guide to their development and use.* (Oxford University Press, Oxford 1989).

44.   A.R. Tarlov, in *Measuring Functioning and Well-Being*, ed. A.L. Stewart and J.E. Ware (Duke University Press, Durham and London, 1992).

45.   J.J. Triano and A.B. Schultz, *Spine* **12** (1987) 561.

46.   M.R. Tuley, C.D. Mulrow, and C.A. McMahan. *J. Clin. Epidemiol.* **44** (1991) 417.

47.   G. Waddell, *Clin. Orthop.* **221** (1987) 110.

48.   G. Waddell and C.J. Main, *Spine* **9** (1984) 204.

49.   G. Waddell, C.J. Main, E.W. Morris, M.D. Paola and I.C.M. Gray, *Spine* **9** (1984) 209.

50.   G. Waddell, C.J. Main, E.W. Morris, et al., *Brit. Med. J.* **284** (1982) 1519.

51.   G. Waddell, D. Somerville, I. Henderson and M. Newton, *Spine* **17** (1992) 617.

52.   J.E. Ware and C.D. Sherbourne, *Med. Care* **30** (1992) 473.

53.   J.E. Ware, K.K. Snow, M. Kosinski and B. Gandek, *SF-36 health survey manual and interpretation guide* (Nimrod Press, Boston, 1993).

54.   I. Wiklund, E. Dimenas and M. Wahl, *Controlled Clinical Trials* **11** (1990) 169.

55.   A.H. Williams, *Brit. Med. J.* **291** (1985) 326.

56.   P.C. Wing, F.J. Wifling and P.J. Kokan, *Clin. Orthop.* **90** (1973) 153.

CHAPTER 3

PAIN SOURCES IN THE LUMBAR SPINE

R.C. Mulholland

1. Introduction

Operations on the lumbar spine are most frequently carried out to relieve pain rather than correct deformity. Inevitably such operations themselves produce tissue injury and distortion, which might in itself cause pain. Yet we hope that such operations may relieve pain, despite being very uncertain as to the causation of pain. A further problem is that we operate at one stage removed from pain, as we assess its severity and significance by observing the disability it produces in the patient. Perhaps not surprisingly the results of much spinal surgery for pain disappoint us.

Although we recognize that pain is an unpleasant experience, with an emotional content, a peripheral source initiating the pain is part of daily experience. The Sherrington-Descarte concept of the protective function of pain is logical and fits in well with our experience of acute pain. However in dealing with long continued or chronic pain there is much change in the neurophysiology. It is necessary to have some understanding of the neurophysiology of pain and recent developments in this field.

1.1. The Gate theory[8]
It is common experience that if one has two pain sources, the lesser pain is hardly felt, the greater pain blocks it. The body has a mechanism to control access of painful stimuli to consciousness, mostly at the spinal level. This is achieved by other stimuli blocking the passage of afferent impulses. The now frequently used transcutaneous nerve stimulators are based on this concept.

1.2. Endorphin concept[9]
The presence within the cerebrospinal fluid (CSF) of naturally occurring anti-pain substances, the endorphins, is well established. The level of these opioid-like substances can be altered. One interesting observation was that the placebo response was endorphin mediated, insofar as it could be reversed by nalorphine. A potent stimulator of endogenous endorphins is exercise, thus explaining its value in chronic pain.

1.3. Neuroplasticity
It has been shown experimentally by Woolf[14] that long continued pain alters the organization of neuronal connections in the spinal cord, facilitating the passage of pain stimuli to the brain. Indeed, in human volunteers he has demonstrated that normal pressure

receptors, if within an area where there is persistent pain stimuli, themselves become wired up centrally to become pain receptors. Clinically we often observe this, as light touch in an area of chronic pain is perceived as painful, commonly referred to as a hypersensitivity of the tissues. This observation has great significance as, obviously, we cannot equate a painful area with the actual pain source.

1.4. Pain sources

A tissue that has no nerves within it will not be able to initiate neuronal impulses of any type. As nerves surround blood vessels perhaps the only non-innervated tissues in the body are the nucleus pulposus of the disc, the lens, and vitreous humour. Clearly, the nerves normally respond to changes in their environment and initiate impulses. Such environmental changes are ill-understood, but appear to produce chemical changes involving prostaglandins and many other chemicals. Modification of these changes is clearly one way to reduce peripheral stimuli, and hence reduce pain. However the nerves themselves can initiate spontaneous impulses, as has been shown by Devor[2]. This is particularly the case if a nerve is injured, and clearly after any operation a large number of nerves in the tissues are so injured. Such an injured nerve undergoes characteristic changes which result in the creation of both false, spontaneous impulses and distortion of normal, transmitted impulses. Indeed, abnormalities of neural processing, in both the peripheral and central nervous system, develop even when the provoking injury is peripheral. Notwithstanding the reality of psychosocial variables in the expression of pain behaviour, there are, therefore, sound neurophysiological reasons for variability in symptoms in different patients if we accept that ectopic neural pacemakers may develop in injured nerves. One further fascinating aspect of Devor's work is that specific strains of rats can be bred which are more likely to develop such neuronal changes after injury than others.

1.5. Nature of pain

The work of Devor[3] and Woolf[15] gives support to the concept that pain may be considered to be of two types: so called physiological pain, transient and clearly protective, and pathological pain, which tends to be chronic, and to have no protective function. It seems likely that this latter pain is a consequence of either altered peripheral receptor and nerve function or a consequence of altered neuronal connections within the spinal cord and central nervous system. It is of interest that opiates and other narcotics are effective in physiological pain, but are not effective in pathological pain. Pathological pain tends to be initiated by minimal stimuli and is more often associated with emotional depression, whereas physiological pain bears a closer relationship to the intensity of the stimulus, and is associated with emotional anxiety rather than depression.

Therefore, when we are considering an operation on the lumbar spine to modify or reduce pain we must be aware that we are attempting to alter the initiating stimulus to a very complex system, the endpoint of which is an emotional experience modified considerably by the outside environment. We must also be aware that surgical injury itself produces neurophysiological changes which may amplify established pain patterns, clearly a very important consideration in repeated back operations in the problem back patient.

2. Pain sources in the lumbar spine: anatomical considerations

All structures in the lumbar spine, other than the nucleus pulposus and the deeper layers of the annulus fibrosus, are potential pain sources insofar as they are innervated. However, anatomical considerations have been somewhat disappointing in terms of their contribution to understanding the nature of back pain. Grossly anatomically abnormal structures are often quite painless, yet pain is often ascribed to tissues where anatomical disruption is minimal. Despite this, it is of value to consider the innervation of the various spinal structures and the possible implications of anatomical disorder and pain initiation.

2.1. Intervertebral disc

It is well established that only the outer few millimetres of the normal disc have any innervation. Pathological discs may develop vascular ingrowth, and very painstaking work by some histologists indicate that nerve tissue accompany these vessels. However the paucity of such nerves would appear to make it unlikely that they are a major pain source, unless one postulates that they are very abnormal nerves and 'fire' inappropriately.

2.2. Facet joints

Because these are diarthrodial joints, and so can develop arthritic changes, they have been regarded since the early part of the century as prime initiators of activity related pain. Unfortunately the pain they produce cannot be identified as a clearly defined syndrome. It seems likely that they may occasionally be a source of an acute episode of back pain, but in longstanding back pain their role is of much less importance.

2.3. Muscles

Muscles are certainly pain sources, anyone who has done excessive and unaccustomed exercise is well aware of the aching pain which follows. Clearly, muscle tears are painful. It seems likely that some acute episodes of back pain following sudden stress are from muscle injury, but recovery is rapid. It is doubtful if, in the non-operated back, muscle pain is significant in the patient with longstanding back pain. Sophisticated EMG studies certainly demonstrate that in a patient with chronic back pain there is considerable alteration in muscle function which of course may be interpreted by the patient as pain. However the very dramatic changes seen on MRI in the muscles of the multi-operated back, raises the suspicion that they may well be a pain source, if only from ischaemia on exercise in these patients.

2.4. Ligaments

Although in other parts of the body (knee, ankle) chronic ligamentous pain is well established and ligaments are appropriately innervated, in the lumbar spine, apart from the outer layer of the annulus, the role of ligaments as a pain source is uncertain. However, if abnormal movement, usually translational, is deemed to be a cause of pain, so called 'instability', then the pain source is presumably the outer layers of the annulus. Certainly the outer annulus can be very sensitive in some patients. MRI scanning sometimes reveals an anterior annular rupture, and in some of these patients the annulus is certainly very tender if palpated through the abdomen. Even in the absence of anterior annular rupture a degenerate disc can be painful if palpated anteriorly.

Interspinous ligaments are often found to be deficient at operations, but no convincing study has shown these finding to be of significance. Although much work has been done concerning the significance of the ilio-lumbar ligament in providing stability, its role as a pain source has not been assessed. The sacro-iliac ligaments are commonly targeted for local injections of irritant materials to produce fibrosis but there is a lack of any evidence for the rationale of this procedure. One suspects that it may achieve success because of pain modulation, as the injections are extremely painful.

2.5. Lumbar fascia

The lumbar fascia is an important structure in the overall function of the spine, transmitting the stabilizing function of the abdominal muscles to the spine. During needling of the spine in the chronic back pain sufferer, the patient may experience pain as the needle goes through the fascia. However, in the normal or relatively normal spine the fascia seems to be quite insensitive. Injury to the fascia occurs in the paravertebral exposure of the spine (Wiltse approach) yet such an approach is not associated with unusual pain, either in the short term or long term.

2.6. Vertebral endplate

The endplate is richly innervated, and endplate changes are a common feature of degenerative disc disease. Work by Shackleford and McNally[10] in the human has shown that disc degeneration leads to abnormal loading of the endplate, a source of pain in diarthrodial joints. Clearly, relatively modest changes may produce significant peaks and troughs of loading over the end-plate, and what is attractive about this concept, is that the grossly degenerate disc, commonly painless, will once again evenly load over the endplate. The frequent association of back pain with a posture associated with high loading, rather than movement, again encourages the concept that much back pain may be load related, rather than movement related. It is hoped that the use of 'pressure profilometry' combined with standard discography may identify the painful disc more precisely.

3. Biochemical considerations

If biomechanics could be said to be the obsession of the seventies and eighties, biochemical considerations are likely to be the obsession of the nineties. In the late eighties Sahl and co-workers[12] identified high levels of phospho-lipase A in the disc, an important enzyme in the pain cascade. Numerous other enzymes have subsequently been identified in disc material, and these are capable of producing significant changes in adjacent nerve roots and, presumably, other structures around the disc such as endplate and annulus. It is attractive to postulate that these chemical mediators of pain are at a high level at certain stages in disc degeneration and produce local inflammation which cause normal movement or loading to be painful. Certainly, the clinical history of some episodes of acute lumbago, (a mild prodromal pain with a very acute onset after trivial physical stimulus, followed by a rapid recovery over a few days and no apparent long term sequelae) fit in with a chemical mediator (akin to an acute capsulitis of the shoulder) rather than a physical injury. Kawakami *et al.* have demonstrated that disc material can induce intra-neural change by chemical means and such changes can be associated with changes within the spinal cord[6].

4. Clinical implications

Clearly, therefore, any of the innervated structures in the lumbar spine may be a pain source. However any investigation of potential pain sources must be preceded by a careful clinical evaluation of the nature of the pain, especially the recognition of the presence of pathological pain. It seems that if the likelihood of modifying this by operative intervention is small, the aim of the clinician is then to identify the physiological pain component. If this can be removed perhaps in time there may be an amelioration of the pathological pain element. Thus we may improve patients pain by appropriate surgical intervention, but cannot remove all pain. Indeed clinical experience suggests that a successful operation in the very pain disabled patient moves them up a grade or two in function, but never alleviates all their pain. A corollary of this is that early intervention by appropriate surgery in disorders known to be associated with the development of chronic pain may be more successful than late intervention.

4.1. Activity-related back pain

Much back pain appears to be related to activity and movement, and it would appear to be almost self-evident that pain produced by movement relates to dysfunction of one or more mobile segments. However, it will be clear from our imperfect understanding of pain described above that normal impulses received by an abnormal neuraxis may produce pain, especially if the pain has the characteristics of pathological pain. A believable concordance between pain experience and the movement generating it encourages the belief that the pain is physiological and intervention to stop or modify movement at that segment may be appropriate. Can we identify those structures in the segment which are the pain sources? Clinical examination can usually identify roughly the site of dysfunction, although lumbo-sacral pain may be referred from the whole of the lumbar spine and even the thoraco-lumbar segments, whereas fascial pain and tenderness, deformity, and asymmetrical movement at other sites in the lumbar spine are more specific. Plain X-rays, CT or MRI may identify pathology which may be relevant but, unfortunately, no imaging will image a pain source, so we cannot be confident that demonstrated pathology is indeed the source of the patient's pain.

5. Clinical investigation of activity-related back pain

The clinical problem that the clinician faces is that if it has been decided that the pain and disability that the patient has is sufficiently significant in social and economic terms to justify consideration of surgical intervention, and that the nature of the pain is such that it is likely to be associated with segmental dysfunction, then the clinician has to identify the segment or segments involved. It must be confessed that knowledge of the nature of this dysfunction is probably rather uncertain. It may be abnormal translation on loading (instability), recognizing that such abnormal movement may be entirely painless, it may be abnormal load patterns over the endplate or facet arthrosis restricted to the segment deemed to be painful. Finally, it may be a chemical inflammation of the disc, rendering normal movement painful. The clinician makes the assumption that either stopping movement of the segment or modifying it will alleviate the pain. It is therefore essential that not only is the symptomatic segment identified, but other actually or potentially symptomatic segments are recognized.

5.1. Identification of painful segments

Clinical identification of a painful segment in the lumbar spine is uncertain. No single clinical finding is conclusive. Local tenderness can be of value and, if forward flexion is proportionately more restricted than lateral flexion, then the lower two segments are more likely to be the pain source. Perhaps the best clinical guide is if a history of radicular pain is obtained then the relevant affected segment may be deduced (*eg*. S1 pain - lumbo-sacral). However it is essential to appreciate that the symptom of low back pain can be produced by lesions from T12 to the sacrum.

Flexion and extension films have a chequered history. The aim is to demonstrate abnormal translation at the suspected level. Not all segmental failure is associated with abnormal translation, and not all painful segments are associated with abnormal translation. If the movement is painful the likelihood is that the patient will not bend enough to demonstrate it. Some surgeons rely on the use of a load, and giving analgesic before the investigation. In patients with spondylolisthesis such films are of value as they can reveal the degree of instability of the segment and guide the surgeon concerning the type of surgery required (decompression alone, or whether it should be combined with fusion).

Facet injections are a popular although somewhat unproven therapy for back pain. It has been established that one cannot identify a specific pattern of pain which can be said to derive from the facet joints. However its use as a diagnostic test to establish level has not been proven. Certainly, if used for this purpose, the local anaesthetic must be placed in the facet joint alone (facet arthrogram), be of a quantity (0.5 ml) to ensure it does not spread, and must not be combined with steroid, which has a systemic effect.

Root block is an important diagnostic and indeed therapeutic manoeuvre. It is essential when using this technique, especially for diagnostic purposes to use no more than 0.5 ml as any more may spread within the psoas and confuse the diagnosis. The other problem of using a larger amount is that it will block the motor fibres; after a 5th-root block patients will have a foot drop, and those with upper roots blocked may have unstable quadriceps. Both of these effects may persist for a few hours and cause them to stay in hospital whereas if smaller amounts are used the diagnostic result, *i.e.* pain relief, is achieved and patients can go home immediately after the injection. The injection clearly must be done under radiological control, contrast should be used to demonstrate where the injection is going, and a hard copy must be kept. The use of a nerve stimulator removes the necessity of penetrating the nerve to confirm position, and in relation to the 1st sacral root, a higher success rate is achieved.

Discography is the most popular technique to establish whether a morphologically abnormal disc is painful and therefore likely to be symptomatic[1,13]. The mechanism of pain production is uncertain; the correlation between the degree of morphological abnormality and pain is poor. However, the results of fusion in patients where the level fused had a painful disc on discography are somewhat better than results when preliminary discography was negative. Fusion of a discographically painless disc achieved a 60% success rate as opposed to an 80% success rate for the painful disc[1]. In the past it was necessary to puncture a number of discs, now it is customary only to puncture discs shown to be abnormal on MRI. Full patient participation is essential, they must be sufficiently alert to distinguish between reproduction of their pain, and just pain. Disc morphology should be evaluated, especially in the adolescent, as significant annular tears can be present despite a normal MRI scan. Pressure measurements are so dependent on needle position that a single measurement is of no value. However the more sophisticated pressure profiles[10] may well be of value.

The use of an anaesthetic injection into the painful disc is said to be of value in establishing whether the disc is the pain source, but my personal experience is that it is uncertain and non-specific. There has been no study to confirm its value.

Perhaps the greatest value of discography is the opportunity it gives the surgeon to evaluate the patient's response to pain and gain insight into how sensitive the spine tissues are and the likelihood that the pain is pathological rather then physiological.

6. External fixation

It would appear logical that if it was believed that movement was the cause of pain and if the movement, and consequently the pain, was stopped by an external fixator, then that would establish that the segment so immobilized was the painful segment. However, the initial enthusiastic report by Esses[4] has been modified and our own experience guarded. It is clear that there is a very high positive response rate, that is to say that external fixation produces significant relief of pain in over 80% of patients. But, subsequent fusion is much less successful. Although fusion success and rigidity of fusion may be a factor, it seems likely that external fixation has some other effect on pain perception over and above immobilization. The nature of this can only be speculated about, but clearly there is some placebo response. However, patients do distinguish between the fixed mode and the unfixed mode on the basis of symptoms alone, so that fixation has some modifying influence on pain. The recent use of the subcutaneous fixator (Simmonds plate) may clarify the situation as it would remove the very externally dramatic nature of the test.

'Soft stabilization' is a term that is used to describe a technique where the spine is fixed in extension using a firm but not rigid artificial ligament. The results seem similar to those of fusion. Such fixation certainly alters endplate loading, but also affects the type of movement, although clearly not abolishing it.

Identification of a pain source is an essential element of any pre-surgical assessment. However, too slavish adherence to the Sherrington concepts of pain, including a failure to recognize the many modifying factors, and the often somewhat tenuous relationship between pain and disability, may lead to inappropriate surgical onslaught on a pain source.

7. References

1.   E. Colhoun, I. McCall, V. Williams and C. Pullicino, *J.Bone Joint Surg.* **70-B**. (1988) 267.

2.   M. Devor, L. Govrin, R. Lippman and K. Angelides, *J. Neurosci.* **13** (1993) 1976.

3.   M. Devor, in *Textbook of Pain* 3rd edn., Eds. P.D. Wall, R. Melzack (Livingstone, London).

4.   S.I. Esses, D.J. Botsford and J.P. Kostuik, *Spine* **14** (1989) 594.

5.   H. Jackson, R. Winkilmann and W. Bichel, *J.Bone Joint Surg.* **48-A** (1966) 1272.

6.   M. Kawakami, J.W. Weinstein and K.F. Spratt, *Spine* **19** (1994) 1789.

7.   W. Lyon, D.J. Hall, R.C. Mulholland and J.K. Webb, in *Lumbar fusion and stabilization*, Eds. K. Yonenobu, K. Ono and Y. Takemitsu, (Springer Verlag).

8.   R. Melzack and P.D. Wall, *Science* **150** (1965) 191.

9.   R. Melzack, *The Puzzle of Pain* (Penguin Education, 1973).

10. I. Shackleford, D.S. McNally and R.C. Mulholland, Abstract, International Society for the Study of the Lumbar Spine Meeting, Seattle, Washington. (1984).

11. M.J.Smythe and V. Wright, *J.Bone Joint Surg.* **40-A** (1958) 1401.

12. J.S. Saal, R.C. Franson, R. Dobrow, J.A. Saal, A.A. White and N. Goldthwaite, *Spine* **15** (1990) 674.

13. T.R. Walsh, J. Weinstein, K. Spratt, T. Lehman, C. Aprile and H. Sayre, *J.Bone Joint Surg.* **72-A** (1990) 1081.

14. C.J. Woolf, C. Molander and M. Reynolds, *Neuroscience* **34** 465.

15. C.J. Woolf, *Trends Neurosci.* **14** (1988) 74.

CHAPTER 4

CHARACTERISATION OF THE INNERVATION TO THE INTERVERTEBRAL DISCS AND ASSOCIATED LIGAMENTS

P.W. McCarthy

1. Introduction

The intervertebral disc (IVD) and posterior longitudinal ligament (PLL) are among the many structures in and around the spinal column which have been implicated as sources of back pain. The basis for this was the possibility that they have some form of innervation. Therefore, the initial research emphasis was on searching for nerve fibres and obvious endings in these tissues. Later this developed into attempts to determine the presence of those nerve fibres which are involved with the perception of pain, namely the nociceptors. In any case, their potential role in the aetiology of back pain has inevitably coloured any research involving these tissues and is encapsulated in statements such as this by Bogduk "… whatever it is in the lumbar spine that causes pain, it must have a nerve supply"[7].

Initial research into the innervation used techniques which have either a poor resolving power, or low specificity (such as heavy metal impregnation and precipitation, intra-vital staining with methylene blue or enzyme reactivity such as with acetylcholinesterase). Such studies were valuable in that they allowed the problem to be identified and gave a wealth of data. The presence of nerves and the more obvious large receptor endings were clearly demonstrated and some indication given of extent of the innervation in these tissues[20,22,24,48,50,52,54]. However, the low specificity of the staining limited any functional interpretation of the results. Further limitations of these techniques arise from their relative lack of selectivity and inability clearly to resolve fine neuronal elements within such highly ordered structures as the IVD (Figure 1). Such problems allowed doubt to be cast on the very existence of the innervation to some structures such as the outer annular fibres of the IVD. Furthermore, it left the area conveniently vague allowing any interpretation of their functional capacity. As a result, this type of study is currently rarely used[11].

1.1. Immunohistochemistry

The main vehicle for studying innervation currently tends to be immunohistochemistry, *i.e.* the use of antibodies, which has been employed extensively. However, like previous staining methods, it also has its problems. The amount of information available about each antibody makes interpretation potentially just as difficult as with the "less refined"

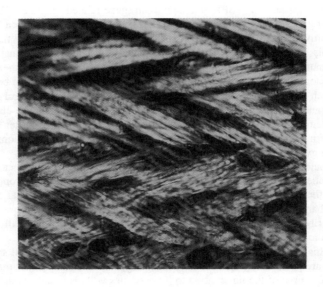

Figure 1. Section of rat IVD (mid to outer annulus fibrosus) stained with haematoxylin. Note the cells which lie in between the interleaving collagen bundles.

methods. Although antibodies are renowned for their specificity of reaction, such specificity is relative. Immunologically similar compounds can react with the same antibody and, as many of the markers used for identifying sub-populations of neurones are small peptides, the potential for cross-reactivity is high. This is referred to as false positive staining. In addition to the potential for false positive staining, some antibodies may not recognise their antigen in certain tissues (false negative) either because it cannot penetrate the structure[45], or because the antigenic site is not available, as found with anti-choline acetyl-transferase antibodies in the same species, until recently[48]. For these reasons, when one refers to the presence of immunoreactivity with an antibody one does so either using the suffix '-like immunoreactivity' (-LI) or '-immunoreactive' (-IR) which acknowledge the possibility of non-specific interaction. This potential for mis-interpretation can be compounded when those antibodies which have been characterised in one species are then used in other species, especially when detailed background studies have not been performed in those species. A further problem, related to this, stems from the fact that immunological similarity does not necessarily equate to functional similarity, even in the same animal.

If an antibody is used successfully to localise a substance in one species then it's reactivity in another species has tended to be accepted as proof of the presence and, on occasion, functional activity of the structures. This has been especially noticeable with respect to the more commonly used antibodies specific to the primary afferent related neuropeptides substance P (SP) and calcitonin gene-related peptide (CGRP). The culmination of their use in a number of species has been the only too common "discovery" of "pain-sensitive fibres". Such links between species are easier to imply than confirm, however. This situation is exacerbated by the paucity of available information directly relating immunohistochemistry (or any other neural stain) to the functional (electrophysiological) characteristics of any neuronal population. There have been attempts to perform such research on primary afferent neurones from the lumbar dorsal root ganglia of rats, cats and guinea pigs[33]. This work has attempted functional sub-classification. However, attempting to relate electrophysiology to any histological marker or group of markers is both difficult and time consuming. Consequently, few populations have been studied to the extent required to be useful in such an interpretation.

One species in which a serious attempt has been made to correlate immunohistochemical characteristics of sensory neurones with their electrophysiological properties is the rat[33,34,35,40,41]. These studies have been limited to the dorsal root ganglia from the lumbar spine. From this it has been hypothesised that tissue whose innervation derives primarily or exclusively from this source may be studied histologically with some confidence as to the functional/electrophysiological interpretation.

Against this background this chapter will now consider in more detail some of the tissues which are potentially important in the aetiology of low back pain, namely the IVD and PLL. The source of the innervation to these tissues will also be discussed.

2. Intervertebral disc

2.1. General features

The general structure and location of the IVD are illustrated in Figure 2. Problems associated with those studies which have used less specific staining techniques can only be appreciated when put into context. The regular organisation of the annular fibrocartilage (stained for clarity in Figure 1) affects the light passing through the tissue. The resulting distortion of the image is greatest at the edge of the annular fibres. Any innervation present tends to lie in the spaces between the annular fibres, *i.e.* the area of greatest distortion, thus increasing the difficulty in resolving detail. Such tissue idiosyncrasies can become insurmountable barriers when studying the fine-filamentous structures associated with the sensory/autonomic terminals *in situ* with heavy metal or the intra-vital stains[24].

It has been shown repeatedly that the central nucleus pulposus of healthy adults is devoid of both vascular and nervous tissue. Even when ingrowing granulation tissue is invading the nucleus in a degenerating IVD it appears largely, if not totally, devoid of nervous tissue[24]. A large proportion of the inner annulus fibrosus also appears devoid of both vascular and nervous tissue. The outer layers of this structure have had varying levels of innervation assigned to them. It is now generally accepted that at least some neuronal tissue is present and may terminate there. The type of innervation which has been regularly studied and discussed is generally primary sensory/afferent in origin or function[13,20,22,24,47,50,54].

There have been some reports of a limited blood supply in the outer annulus fibrosus of both adult animals and apparently healthy humans (those with no obvious back

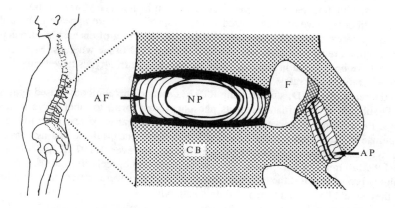

Figure 2. Orientation of the IVD within the body. The lamellae of the annulus fibrosus (AF) become more tightly packed in the posterior IVD. The other structures which limit rotational movement of the IVD are the zygapophyseal or facet joints (one of these is labelled: AP). Nerve roots exit the spinal canal via the intervertebral foramen (F).

pathology) up to 70 years of age[8,25]. This vascularisation is known to become much more extensive, and therefore noticeable, in pathological tissue. As the vascular system and sympathetic vasomotor system appear to be inextricably linked, it is only to be expected that an autonomic nerve supply may also be present. The extent of such a nerve supply has not been studied in any great detail. However, it has been indicated by the presence of neuropeptide-Y-like (NPY-LI) fibres in normal annulus fibrosus[1]. However, simply finding NPY-LI in pathological tissue and referring to it as of sympathetic origin may be erroneous. There is an up-regulation of the expression of this neuropeptide by sensory neurones in neuropathology which may lead to NPY-LI being present in afferent nerve fibres[27]. Therefore, the presence of immunoreactivity to the enzymes involved in noradrenaline synthesis, dopamine-beta hydroxylase (DBH)-LI, or tyrosine hydroxylase (TH)-LI, is usually taken as confirmation that the adrenergic limb of the autonomic nervous system is present. The possible presence of NPY-LI and TH-LI fibres on the surface of the rat lumbar IVD has been indicated[1], however no detail of where (posterior/anterior), how much or whether these antigens were co-localised has been presented. Therefore, as stated above, this region has not yet been extensively studied using markers for the sympathetic adrenergic nervous system.

2.2. Innervation: myelinated fibres

The sensory, primary afferent innervation has been studied by many non-specific techniques. The poor resolution inherent in earlier techniques, compounded by the arrangement and highly refractive nature of the tissue, made the initial findings vague and contentious with few receptors being illustrated; although many were reported. Pan-specific antibodies have also been used in this respect[16,18]. There appears to be a direct relationship between size of animal species and the reporting of encapsulated receptors. Larger Pacinian receptors have been found in human IVD tissue whereas, Meissner-like receptors have been found in humans, dogs and rats and Ruffini-types have being reported in humans, rabbits and rats[11,12,16,18,20,22,24,36, 47,50,52,54].

In the rat lumbar IVD, studies using RT97 (a monoclonal antibody raised against the 200 kD subunit of neurofilament in its phosphorylated form) to label nerve fibres and endings, *i.e.* myelinated nerves[33,35], showed that they appear to be restricted to the outer 1-2 laminae of the annulus at their deepest[42]. Few large encapsulated endings have been found in or around the rat IVD using this antibody. However, RT97-IR has been shown to label the full range of encapsulated receptors in rat tissue, including skin[49]. Therefore, it is highly probable that if the larger encapsulated receptors were present in the rat lumbar IVD, they would have been found with this antibody.

There appears to be a consensus between early and recent studies with respect to the relationship between encapsulated receptors and the anterior annulus. This has been reported in a variety of species using either pan-neuronally specific antibodies such as PGP9.5 and Protein S-100[16,18], neurofilament antibodies specific for myelinated fibres such as RT97[49], or silver-based staining techniques. A degree of spatial variation in density of those larger encapsulated endings has been reported, with the larger, encapsulated endings in the rat, dog and human being located mainly in or on the anterior or antero-lateral aspect of the IVD close to the cartilage-end plate[12,18,24,36,42]. Such a juxtaposition between receptors and IVD/vertebrae would suggest a proprioceptive function and postural feedback control. This system could monitor the degree of stretching occurring on the anterior surface, which would relate to extension of the spine. However, the type of the natural stimulus and whether the information can be used in posture control is still debatable.

One further piece of the puzzle is known. In a retrograde labelling study of the innervation to the annulus of thoracolumbar discs in the dog, the primary afferent component to this IVD was found to originate from the two dorsal root ganglia rostral and the two caudal to the injected IVD[13]. This would appear to put some limit on the precision expected from the nervous system. However, no mention of the size or type of cell labelled was presented and so the distribution of that small contribution from the myelinated population can not be resolved further at present. The question of capability which needs to be resolved is whether the myelinated population of afferents can only give information of use in general postural control or has it the ability to lead to simple segmental reflexes, each of which could affect muscle activity involved in the stability of the spinal column. Such information will be crucial to our determining the capabilities of this component of the innervation. However, for the answers to questions such as these we will, of necessity, have to await results of more direct studies, such as those proposed for IVDs[11] similar to those previously performed on facet joints by Cavanaugh's group and others[5,14,54].

2.3. *Peptidergic innervation: Chemical coding*

There is a growing trend towards the 'chemical-coding' of the neurones in any tissue. With the lack of direct evidence of a functional capacity, this type of study develops a framework around which research into the functional nature can be undertaken. Chemical coding relies on the visible presence of antigenic markers in the peripheral fibres and the ability to determine co-localisation within nerve fibres. This may not always be possible, especially with sparsely innervated tissue, as it can only be performed adequately at the electron microscope level or when cell bodies are available for study. However, a sound knowledge of the combinations which exist in a species makes some extrapolation possible from data gathered from nerve fibres at the light microscope level. As a further note of caution, when interpreting chemical coding one should remember that it will probably change between species, as will the any functional significance, for example in the afferent nerve supply of rats CGRP-LI can easily be found without SP-LI whereas in the guinea pig they are almost totally co-localised in primary afferents.

The density, relative location and type of smaller diameter thinly myelinated and unmyelinated peptide-LI containing neurones have been most extensively reported. The majority of these studies, however, have given only qualitative details. Such studies run the risk of drawing erroneous conclusions which later, more detailed studies find difficult to overturn. Those fibres which have been described are varicose (sometimes described as a string of pearls) and branched, with no obviously encapsulated terminal structures, where these have been looked for.

2.4. *Peptidergic innervation: Substance P*

Substance P-like immunoreactivity (SP-LI) was initially not found in human annulus fibrosus[32], although later, more thorough studies found a sparse innervation in the outer laminae[12]. Vasoactive intestinal peptide (VIP), SP and CGRP -LIs were all reported in rat IVD tissue, with no details of method or antibodies used, just poor quality photomicrographs[51]. However, since these initial studies, more detailed and robust work has been reported with quantitative details being described for rats[37]. The degree of quantification in many reports tends to be related to size and availability of the tissue. Therefore, studies involving the lower vertebrates (*eg*. rats and rabbits) tend to survey the extent, amount and any obvious terminal structures present in the innervation, whereas many human studies may only be able to indicate the presence and relative proportion.

SP-LI has been shown in trailing fibres which have the typical varicose appearance and extend into the outer 5-6 layers of the annulus fibrosus[37]. The distribution of SP is relatively uniform, if sparse, around the IVD. Some finely branched endings were found, along with varicose fibres which followed convoluted and tortuous paths near their endings[12,37]. Varicosities in the fibre terminals lie in close proximity to the cells which reside in the matrix between collagen bundles (Figure 3). Whether this is a consequence of the highly organised structure or some functional juxtaposition is unknown at present. However, the smaller number of fibres present would suggest a limited action, especially if the SP can be protected from endogenous enzymatic degradation by endopeptidases[2,3] and prevented from diffusing. The positioning of SP fibres in the rat would suggest some role for this peptide in matrix repair or production. This idea was tested using concentrations

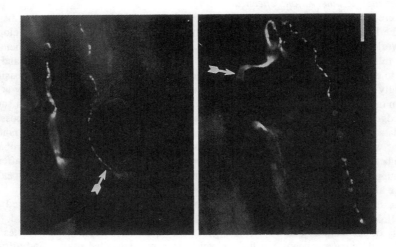

Figure 3. SP-LI varicose fibres. The left photomicrograph shows varicosities around a cell body (arrow). The right photomicrograph shows a SP-LI fibre following a tortuous path between the collagen bundles of the outer annulus fibrosus (arrow at the start). Scale bar 10 μm.

of SP which would be expected in the annulus fibrosus on the cells which produce proteoglycans[2]. Both the proliferation and proteoglycans production were increased significantly in the presence of SP (especially in the presence of endopeptidase inhibitor). This SP activity clearly suggests a role for the nociceptor peptides in a response to repair damage. However, this does not preclude the potential for such peptides to have a role in the constant maintenance, if not homeostasis, of the IVD. The potential for such a role becomes more apparent if one also considers the reduced proteoglycan synthesis and proliferation of matrix cells[10] with ageing alongside the finding sensitivity to the sensory peptides in the periphery decreases with age[28]. It may be that there is a relationship between the decrease in sensitivity, decreased matrix formation and slow degeneration of the outer elements of the IVD seen with age. An extrapolation of the same hypothesis in respect to pathology was used to describe the generation of scoliosis, based on the observation that more SP-LI was present on the thicker side of scoliotic IVDs[46].

2.5. Peptidergic innervation: Calcitonin gene-related peptide

The innervation by CGRP-LI fibres in the rat appears to be as extensive, though more dense, than that of SP-LI[39,42]. This is not surprising as these two immunoreactivities generally co-localise in this species with >95% of the lumbar SP-LI containing primary afferent neurones also containing CGRP-LI[33,35]. CGRP-LI primary afferents, on the other hand, do not all contain SP-LI (about 50% of CGRP-LI dorsal root ganglion cells contain SP-LI). Therefore, one would expect to find more CGRP-LI fibres if a mixed afferent population were present. Some of these CGRP-LI fibres are also labelled with RT97-IR showing that they are myelinated afferents[42]. This might suggest that, in the rat at least, some of the CGRP-LI fibres may form part of the more obviously mechano-receptive fibres surrounding the IVD.

The 'unmyelinated' (RT97-IR negative, C-fibres) afferents in the rat, which penetrate deeper (up to 6 lamellae) into the annulus, may be split into two populations: CGRP-LI only and CGRP-LI co-localised with SP-LI[37,38,39]. This suggests at least two sub-populations of fine afferents may be present and raises the question of an independent role for CGRP in the annulus fibrosus to match that of SP discussed above.

Apart from any independent function of CGRP, this peptide is also known to potentiate indirectly the activity of SP. Such an action derives from the competition between these peptides for degradation by the endopeptidase enzyme. As mentioned above, endopeptidase inhibition significantly increases the activity of SP on cell proliferation and proteoglycan synthesis, indicating that if the CGRP acts in this way SP would be much more effective as a stimulant of this cellular activity. CGRP and SP are co-localised and would therefore be co-released from the neurones. This would put the CGRP in the most effective place, both temporally and spatially, to compete with SP for the degrading enzyme[15]. Although SP can increase activity of fibroblasts, neither CGRP or VIP have shown consistent effects on fibroblast proliferation, however this interesting area is open to further investigation.

CGRP and SP also have a number of vascular effects, which may have consequences in the outer annulus fibrosus. As mentioned earlier, the limited vascularisation appears to be present in the same regions as the innervation[8,25]. CGRP has been shown to be vasodilatory in a variety of tissues[21]. SP on the other hand compliments the CGRP vasodilation in injury by causing extravasation of fluid and mast cell degranulation. CGRP is also capable of causing neutrophil accumulation in tissue[9], thus completing the inflammation. An increase in nociceptor sensitivity could also result from excess SP release[53]. These activities may be initiated on stimulation of a tissue innervated by nociceptors containing these peptides, which in turn may be sensitised by the SP they release. As part of an acute healing reaction (neurogenic vasodilatation and neurogenic inflammation, Lewis triple response) they are invaluable, so it should come as no surprise that the outer regions of the annulus is the only part to have a demonstrable healing (fibrosis) reaction after trauma[19].

When considering the potentially direct actions of CGRP on the annulus fibrosus, independently of SP, one should look to the activity found in other tissues. The most obvious action of CGRP is that of vasodilatation. A similar action to that found for CGRP in gastric mucosa[21] could be of potential use in the IVD. Acid stimulation of chemically sensitive nociceptors leads to CGRP release resulting in vasodilatation. In a similar way, acid may build-up in the annulus fibrosus because the flow of waste products from the nucleus pulposus is mainly via the annulus fibrosus[44]. It may be postulated that the limited annular vasculature may have a role in preventing the waste products building up and becoming a toxic environment for cells in the outer annulus[38]. An outline of the potential role for this part of the innervation in the outer annulus is given in Figure 4.

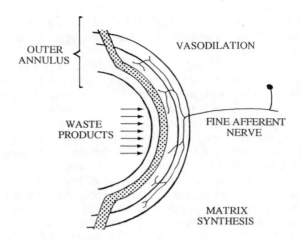

Figure 4. Schematic diagram showing the possible roles for the fine afferent (peptidergic) nerve fibres found in the outer annulus fibrosus. CGRP release could lead to vasodilation in the control of the environment and SP could affect matrix synthesis. In this scenario, the stimulus for increased release would be local pH (or lactate) change caused by the waste products constantly issuing from the deeper tissue.

2.6. Peptidergic innervation: Other peptides

VIP-LI fibres have also been located inside and on the posterior surface of the annulus[1,51]. These have a similar characteristics to SP-LI and CGRP-LI, being varicose in nature. No real detail is currently available about the distribution density or their density relative to other markers. As there is little if any co-localisation between VIP and CGRP-LI in the rat lumbar primary afferent supply[33], one can only postulate that this may be a further separate functional component of the innervation. However, so little is known about this population of afferents that their role in this tissue cannot be speculated on at present. As with CGRP, VIP is also a vasodilator[21]. However, its activity with respect to the fine afferent nerves has not been studied extensively.

Although looked for, immunoreactivity to the neuropeptides enkephalin[30] or somatostatin (SOM) has not yet been reported in the annulus fibrosus. My own studies, using two separate antibodies to SOM on tissue from rat and guinea pig, have been unable to detect SOM-LI fibres. However, this may not be the case in other species.

2.7. Capsaicin studies

Capsaicin is the pungent constituent of hot peppers (Capsicum minimum) which first stimulates then desensitises and degenerates polymodal nociceptors in a number of mammalian species[26]. The capsaicin sensitivity of the primary afferents containing both SP-LI and CGRP-LI (polymodal nociceptors) in rat and guinea pig is well known. The vast majority of nerve fibres containing SP-LI and CGRP-LI are degenerated following treatment of the animal with capsaicin[26]. In these species capsaicin appears selectively to denervate skin and visceral tissues of the polymodal nociceptors. The sensitivity of the innervation to the IVD has been shown in tissue from the guinea-pig lumbar region[43]. This confirms the presence of polymodal nociceptors in the IVD of this species. The corresponding VIP-LI and RT97-IR populations to the same region were unaffected by capsaicin, supporting the supposition that they comprise functionally separate populations.

3. Posterior longitudinal ligament

3.1. General

The posterior longitudinal ligament (PLL) is a continuous spinal ligament which extends the length of the spinal column[17]. It comprises 3 layers: The upper (most posterior) ligamentous layer is more or less continuous from vertebra to vertebra in man and other species which have been studied. The lower (more anterior) ligamentous layer only traverses the vertebral body, fusing at both ends of the vertebra with the cartilage-end plate regions. The neurovascular layer is sandwiched between the two ligamentous layers. The basic shape of the lumbar PLL is denticulate (Figure 5), with the broadened region being over the IVD[17,29,30]. Gross interspecies differences include the thickness and the degree of adhesion between the upper and lower ligamentous components. In rat, these components are strongly adhering, however, in larger species they can be separated more easily[29] (unpublished observations). In humans, the upper PLL ligament can be lifted clear of the IVD where it crosses it[17].

A notable change occurs with respect to the arrangement of the collagen fibres within the PLL as it is stretched, *i.e.* the spine is flexed. The orientations of the collagen bundles in the PLL become more aligned towards the longitudinal axis[4]. Such a change would be

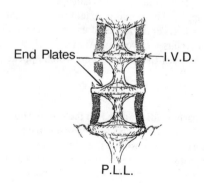

Figure 5. Arrangement of the PLL along the lumbar spine of the rat. The inferior part of the ligament fuses with each end-plate whereas the superior part appears continuous along the length of the spinal column.

perfect for the activation of any proprioceptors embedded in the tissue.

The superficial aspect of the posterior ligament takes on the form of a connective tissue membrane at its posterior border. This membrane appears to envelop the dura mater[29]. In larger species there are noticeable ligamentous connections between the dura mater and PLL (ligaments of Hoffman) which restrict absolute rostro-caudal movement. Some of these connections may help carry the branches of the sinuvertebral nerve which are said to innervate the dura mater[17].

3.2. Innervation

The innervation of the PLL originates from the branches of the sinuvertebral nerve at that vertebral segment and those more rostral and caudal via the ascending and descending branches. In two detailed acetylcholinesterase studies[29,30] the extent of this innervation was documented for the rat lumbar spine. Two levels of innervation were noted over the IVD, the upper ligament being supplied sparsely in contrast to the lower (over the posterior IVD). Varicose fibres were in the majority, yet a number of non-varicose fibres were also evident. The supply to the upper ligament followed a rostro-caudal course passing over the IVD to suggest a similarly organised innervation to that of the IVD (*i.e.* not a truly segmentally arranged input of information). The two main rostro-caudal nerve fibres (one on each side in the rat) ran lateral to the mid-line of the PLL, alongside the edge and its vascular supply in the mid-vertebral level, and crossed over the PLL at the level of the IVD. The plexus over the posterior IVD showed the greatest density of fibres. These formed a network with no obvious orientation to the fibres. In contrast, the fibres of the PLL body (over the vertebral body) showed an approximate rostro-caudal alignment.

3.3. Autonomic innervation

The sinuvertebral nerve has a component of the ventral ramus communicans which could supply some autonomic nerves to this tissue. Furthermore, the vascular supply, which originates from the segmental lumbar arterial supply and basivertebral veins, would also carry an autonomic supply. The possible extent of the adrenergic component of the autonomic nervous system was recently revealed using DBH-LI in the rat lumbar PLL[23]. This confirms and greatly extends the work of Ahmed *et al.* who used NPY-LI and TH-LI[1]. Imai *et al.* gave more detail of the distribution, which appears to follow the vascular system[23].

3.4. Sensory innervation

In contrast to the IVD, early studies agreed on the presence of an extensive innervation to this tissue. In addition, for the PLL and other posterior spinal ligaments, there have been many reports of larger, encapsulated endings such as Ruffini and Pacinian corpuscles[11,17], slowly adapting and rapidly adapting mechanoreceptors, respectively. However, less detailed studies have generally been performed on the PLL compared with the IVD. The general feature for both animal and human sensory innervation is the capacity for fibres to travel from the sensory ganglion over at least one IVD into adjacent segments of PLL before terminating[17,29,30]. The presence of a myelinated afferent component has been intimated.

Early immunohistochemical studies showed the presence of SP-LI in human PLL from over the IVD region[31,32]. The earlier report also suggested no enkephalin (ENK) -LI was present[31]. In the rat, the SP-LI was at its greatest density in the tissue overlying the posterior IVD under the upper PLL component[37,43]. This is consistent with the acetylcholinesterase studies[29,30], though no quantitative details of the SP-LI innervation in the PLL are available. The maximum extent of the SP-LI innervation could be estimated by looking at the recent study of CGRP-LI in the PLL of rats[22]. In this elegant study, the dorsal root ganglia of the lumbar spine were shown to be the primary source of the CGRP-LI innervation to the PLL. They showed that CGRP-LI fibres could terminate in the PLL outside their segment of origin. Their experiment also highlighted that CGRP-LI nerve fibres could use a number of routes to reach the PLL. One of these, which was not considered but could result in the small residual innervation, is that from the dura mater which has a link (ligamentous and neuronal) with the PLL. This may be the reason that some residual innervation was present after denervation. Imai *et al.* claimed that they were revealing the nociceptor population using CGRP-LI[23]. This is not necessarily the correct interpretation because CGRP-LI may be found in myelinated primary afferents, including motor afferents, *i.e.* it is not necessarily specific to nociceptors[33]. However, this is the case when used alone. Further evidence for the supposition that CGRP-LI may be found in non-nociceptors comes from the finding that, in some tissues, a small residual CGRP-LI nerve fibre population may still be present after capsaicin treatment. The demonstration of CGRP-LI in unmyelinated fibres within the tissue[22] can also not be used to support this as some thinly-myelinated sensory fibres may lose their myelination on entering a tissue. However, support for their supposition may be found from the presence of nociceptors in PLL from the guinea-pig lumbar spine which has been suggested in a preliminary report of the susceptibility of many of the CGRP-LI and SP-LI fibres to capsaicin[43]. In the same report there was also a lack of effect of this agent shown on the VIP-LI, NPY-LI and RT97-IR innervations. This would support the presence of nociceptors and put this into context with a variety of other potential sub-populations of neurones innervating these tissues. This factor illustrates the similarity between these tissues and those of the rest of the body; *i.e.* nociceptors are but one population of primary afferent fibre, probably the most ubiquitous.

In the guinea-pig, the SP-LI innervation (which co-localises with CGRP-LI) was extensive in the body of the PLL. This innervation followed the rostro-caudal alignment seen in acetylcholinesterase studies, and was noticeably varicose[43]. A further feature was the capsaicin sensitivity of 95% of this innervation. In other viscera from the same animals (taken as controls) the SP-LI was completely removed, which suggests that a further population of SP-LI/CGRP-LI fibres are present other than the polymodal nociceptors.

4. Conclusions

From this information, it may be possible to surmise some of the roles which the afferent nerve supply plays in these tissues. The large encapsulated receptors (proprioceptors) on the anterior and antero-lateral annulus fibrosus (Figure 6) could have a role in feedback control during spinal extension, the lateral receptors monitoring lateral

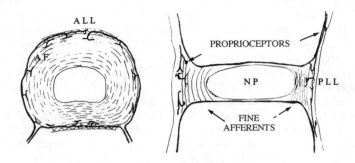

Figure 6. A transverse (left) and sagittal (right) view of the IVD and ligaments showing the positions of proprioceptors and fine (peptidergic) afferents. The uniform supply around the IVD of the latter and the localised arrangement of the former are highly suggestive of independent roles.

deviation during this process. The myelinated component of the PLL innervation, having slowly adapting and rapidly adapting receptors, could report detail about spinal flexion. Receptors with these properties could relay data concerning rate and degree of change in stretch in the tissue. The fact that the innervation is not truly segmental may indicate that these data are used to give an overall appreciation of degrees of flexion and extension, and are not involved with the changes on a segment to segment level. This relates well with preliminary data from studies of lumbar vertebral movement using videofluoroscopy (M. Kondracki, personal communication) which have shown that the patterns of individual vertebral motion during flexion of the spine are more random than regular, even though the overall flexion is smooth.

The peptidergic supply, probably has a trophic effect on the tissue itself, rather than just being involved in some form of segmental reflex control. As previously mentioned, SP-LI fibres appear to affect matrix formation in the outer annulus fibrosus, however, this may not be limited to the IVD as SP-LI and CGRP-LI have also been found in bone and other related tissues[6]. It may be that the supply of nutrients to the central regions of the IVD takes some SP/CGRP along with it, which may help maintain synthesis of matrix in the deeper regions of the IVD. CGRP, which is present in greater quantity, and VIP are both vasodilators. The importance of these peptides to the regulation of blood flow in this region has yet to be investigated. Either way, if the regulatory function of the peptidergic supply is subject to degeneration with age and is increased with pathology[28,46] it might explain the changes seen during these times and go some way to prevention in the future.

5. References

1.   M. Ahmed, A. Bjurholm, M. Kreicbergs and M. Schultzberg, *Spine* **18** (1993) 268.

2. I.K. Ashton and S.M. Eisenstein, *Spine* **21** (1996) 421.
3. I.K. Ashton and S.M. Eisenstein, in *Lumbar Spine Disorders: Current Concepts*, eds. R.M. Aspden and R.W. Porter (World Scientific, London, 1995).
4. R.M. Aspden, *Clin. Anat.* **5** (1992) 372.
5. A. Avramov, J.M. Cavanaugh, A. Cuneyt Ozaktay, T. . Getchell and A.I. King, *J. Bone Joint Surg.* **74-A** (1992) 1464.
6. A. Bjurholm, A. Kreicbergs, E. Brodin and M. Schultzberg, *Peptides* **9** (1988) 165.
7. N. Bogduk, *Spine* **8** (1983) 286.
8. K. Brunner and J. Frewein, *Anat. Histol. Embryol.* **18** (1989) 76.
9. T.L. Buckley, S.D. Brain, M. Rampart and T.J. Williams, *Br. J. Pharmacol.* **103** (1991) 1515.
10. J.A. Buckwalter, *Spine* **20** (1995) 1307.
11. J.M. Cavanaugh, S. Kallakuri and A. Cuneyt Ozaktay, *Spine* **20** (1995) 2080.
12. M.H. Coppes, E. Marani, R.T.W.M. Thomeer, M. Oudega and G.J. Groen, *Lancet* **336** (1990) 189.
13. W.B. Forsyth and N.G. Ghoshal, *Anat. Record* **208** (1984) 57.
14. R.G. Gillette, R.C. Kramis and W.J. Roberts, *Pain* **54** (1993) 85.
15. P. Le Greves, F. Nyberg, L. Terenius and T. Hokfelt, *Eur. J. Pharmacol.* **115** (1985) 309.
16. M. Gronblad, J.N. Weinstein and S. Santavirta, *Acta Orthop. Scand.* **62** (1991) 614.
17. G.J. Groen, B. Baljet, J. Drukker, *Am. J. Anat.* **18** (1990) 282.
18. M. Guillot, H. Pionchon, J. Pialat, B. Bancel and B. Galtier, *Revue du Rhumatisme et des Maladies Osteo Articulaires* **55** (1988) 421.
19. D. Hampton, G. Laros, R. McCarron and D. Franks, *Spine* **14** (1989) 398.
20. C. Hirsch, B-E. Inglemark and M. Miller, *Acta Orthop. Scand.* **33** (1963) 1.
21. P. Holzer and P.H. Guth, *Circ. Res.* **68** (1991) 100.
22. L. Horackova and L. Malinovsky, *Folia Morphol. (Prague)* **35** (1987) 390.
23. S. Imai, S. Hukuda and T. Maeda, *Spine* **20** (1995) 2086.
24. H.C Jackson II, R.K. Winkelmann and W.H. Bickel, *J. Bone Joint Surg.* **48-A** (1966) 1272.
25. K. Jamiolkowska, *Folia Morphol. (Warsz.)* **40** (1981) 363.
26. G. Jancso, *Exp. Physiol.* **77** (1992) 405.
27. H. Kashiba, K. Noguchi, Y. Ueda and E. Senba, *Peptides* **15** (1994) 411.
28. Z. Khalil, V. Ralevic, M. Bassirat, G. J. Dusting and R.D. Helme, *Brain Res.* **641** (1994) 265.
29. Y. Kojima, T. Maeda, R. Arai and K. Shichikawa, *J. Anat.* **169** (1990) 237.
30. Y. Kojima, T. Maeda, R. Arai and K. Shichikawa, *J. Anat.* **169** (1990) 247.
31. Y. Konttinen, M. Gronblad, I. Antti-Poika, S. Seitsalo, S. Santavirta, M. Hukkanen and J.M. Polak, *Spine* **15** (1990) 383.
32. O. Korkala, M. Gronblad, P. Liesi and E. Karaharju, *Spine* **10** (1985) 156.

33.   S.N. Lawson, in *Neurobiology of Nociceptors*, eds F. Cervero and C. Belmonte (1995)

34.   S.N. Lawson, P.W. McCarthy and E. Prabhakar, *J. Comp. Neurol.* **365** (1996) 355.

35.   S.N. Lawson, M.J. Perry, E. Prabhakar and P.W. McCarthy, *Brain Res. Bullet.* **30** (1993) 239.

36.   J. Malinsky, *Acta Anat.* **38** (1959) 96.

37.   P.W. McCarthy, *Acta Orthop. Scand.* **64** (1993) 664.

38.   P.W. McCarthy, *Euro. J. Chiropractic* **41** (1993) 21.

39.   P.W. McCarthy, B. Carruthers, D. Martin and P. Petts, *Spine* **16** (1991) 653.

40.   P.W. McCarthy and S.N. Lawson, *Neurosci.* **28** (1989) 745.

41.   P.W. McCarthy and S.N. Lawson, *Neurosci.* **34** (1990) 623.

42.   P.W. McCarthy, P. Petts and A. Hamilton, *J. Anat.* **180** (1990) 15.

43.   P.W. McCarthy and H. Sann, *Neuropeptides* **24** (1993) 201.

44.   K. Ogata and L.A. Whiteside, *Spine* **6** (1981) 211.

45.   S. Rhalmi, L'H. Yahia, N. Newman and M. Isler, *Spine* **18** (1993) 264.

46.   S. Roberts, in *Lumbar Spine Disorders: Current Concepts*, eds. R.M. Aspden and R.W. Porter (World Scientific, London, 1995).

47.   P.G. Roofe, *Arch. Neurol. Psychiat.* **44** (1940) 100.

48.   H. Sann, P.W. McCarthy, M. Mader and M. Schemann, *Neurosci. Letts.* **198** (1995) 17.

49.   H. Sann, P.W. McCarthy, G. Jancso and F.-K. Pierau, *Cell Tiss. Res.* **282** (1995) 155.

50.   D.L. Stilwell, *Anat. Rec.* **125** (1956) 139.

51.   J. Weinstein, W. Claverie and S. Gibson, *Spine* **13** (1988) 1344.

52.   G. Wiberg, *Acta Orthop. Scand.* **19** (1949) 211.

53.   T. Yamashita, J.M. Cavanaugh, C. Ozaktay, A.I. Avramov, T.V. Getchell and A.I. King, *J. Orthop. Res.* **11** (1993) 205.

54.   H. Yoshizawa, J.P. O'Brien, W.T. Smith and M. Trumper, *J. Pathol.* **132** (1980) 95.

CHAPTER 5

THE ROLE OF THE BLOOD SUPPLY IN LUMBAR SPINE DISORDERS

I.L.H. Reichert, I.D. McCarthy and S.P.F. Hughes

1. Introduction

The underlying pathology and pathophysiology of lumbar spine disorders is poorly understood and one area requiring investigation is the blood supply to the structures of the lumbar spine.

The structures of the lumbar spine show differences in normal blood flow and perfusion. The intervertebral discs are the largest avascular structures of the body and their nourishment by diffusion was investigated by Urban *et al.*[1]. The two main parts of the intervertebral disc, the annulus fibrosus and the nucleus pulposus, have to be treated separately, as there is some blood flow in the annulus fibrosus[2]. The vertebral bodies consist of cancellous bone encapsulated in a thin shell of cortical bone at the sides and the vertebral endplates cranial and caudal.

The avascular nucleus pulposus receives its nutrition through the annulus fibrosus and the vertebral endplates. Experimental work undertaken by Ogata and Whiteside[3] on the canine lumbar spine has shown that the vertebral endplate is the dominant region for exchanging fluid with the nucleus pulposus. Small molecules such as glucose, are transported through a process of diffusion, whereas a 'mechanical pumping' effect caused by movements of the spine is needed to transport larger molecules, such as proteins[4].

2. Anatomy

2.1. Blood supply to the vertebral body

The vertebral body can be seen as an abbreviated long bone. Brookes[5] observed that both the vertebral body and long bones have similarities in their vascular structure. A lumbar vertebra receives its blood supply from the paired lumbar arteries, which arise from the posterior wall of the abdominal aorta. Each artery courses horizontally around the mid part of the vertebral body. The relation of these arteries and their branches to the periosteum of the vertebral body is described by Crock *et al.*[6] as laying 'on' and not embedded 'in'. He went on to describe the following branches that are given off by the lumbar arteries supplying the vertebral body from anterior: the centrum branches, ascending branches and descending branches. The centrum branches pierce to the intraosseus centrum of the vertebra, ascending and descending branches course towards the 'metaphyses' of the vertebral body. There are anastomoses between the ascending and

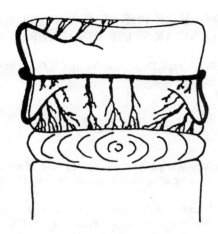

Figure 1. Diagram of the arterial supply to a lumbar vertebral body seen in the midcoronal plane

descending branches of the lumbar arteries on the anterior and posterior surfaces of the anterior longitudinal ligament in front of the intervertebral disc. A similar system of blood supply to the vertebra is described on its posterior aspect. The anterior spinal canal branches arising off the lumbar arteries form arcades on the posterior surfaces of the vertebrae, supplying it with centrum branches and ascending and descending branches. Longitudinal anastomoses occur between the ascending and descending branches on the posterior surface of the intervertebral disc, but not as numerous as on the anterior aspect. Inside the vertebral body the centrum branches form an arterial grid in its middle, from which vertically oriented branches pass to the middle thirds of the vertebral endplates. The 'metaphyseal' branches supply the anterior lateral and posterior lateral parts of the vertebral bodies and contribute vertical branches to the endplates (Figure 1).

2.2. Blood supply of the vertebral endplate

Injection studies on adult dogs *in vivo* led Crock *et al.*[6] to the following description of the vascularity of the vertebral endplate. The vertebral endplate is supplied by a capillary bed sourced by the centrum and metaphyseal arteries, branches of the paired lumbar arteries. Although segmental supply of the vertebral endplate by arteries from different extraosseous vessels has been observed, intraosseous anastomoses between small arteries are present. Therefore the bone-disc interface has been shown to have a continuous capillary bed.

Overlying the area of the nucleus pulposus the capillary terminations are discoid and are described by Crock *et al.*[6] as appearing like "suckers on the tentacles of an octopus". Recent scanning electron microscopic examination of the vertebral endplates in the rabbit by Oki *et al.*[7] has shown loops of arteriola, which the investigators describe as vascular buds. The loop structure, seen as well in the renal glomeruli, might be important for the transport of material into the disc. In the region of the annulus fibrosus the density of capillaries is lower than in the area related to the nucleus pulposus.

2.3. Venous drainage

Subchondrally, a complex postcapillary network of venules has been described close to the disc-bone interface[8]. Drainage follows into a large subarticular horizontal collecting vein and further into the anterior internal vertebral venous plexus within the spinal canal (Figure 2).

Saywell *et al.*[9] have shown that it is possible to observe the endplate veins in patients at levels remote from the site of disc pathology using magnetic resonance imaging (MRI). Anastomoses through fine marrow veins lead to the basi-vertebral vein in the centre of the vertebral body, which drains as well into the internal vertebral venous plexus. The emerging venous plexus radicles surround the lumbar nerve roots. Crock[10] showed that intraoperative filling of the venous plexus is an indication of successful operative decompression of a nerve root. Work by Breschet[11] in the early nineteenth century pointed out that there are no valves in the internal venous plexuses, allowing the direction of flow to be altered. Adjacent bones of the vertebral column are connected by large extra-osseous veins into which the nutrient veins drain. Thus, as Brookes[5] observed, the vertebral column can be regarded as a vascular unit.

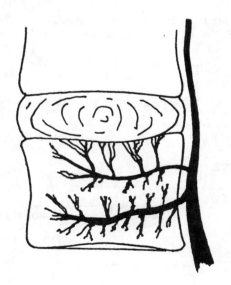

Figure 2. Diagram of the venous system of a lumbar vertebral body seen in the midsagittal plane.

3. Physiology

Clinically there is no generally accepted method of measuring regional blood flow to the skeletal system in the human subject. Hughes *et al.*[12] undertook experimental work in large animals which gave a detailed account of regional blood flow to the annulus fibrosus and the adjacent vertebral endplates using the indicator fractionation tecinnique with radiolabelled microspheres.

The radiolabelled microsphere technique is still regarded as the standard method for measuring experimentally the regional distribution of blood flow in most organs. Their application to the measurement of bone blood flow has been reviewed by Tothill[13]. Microspheres are injected into the heart and are trapped in the microcirculation. Their distribution is in proportion to the cardiac output to that region. Withdrawal of blood at a known flow rate from a suitable artery while the microspheres are being injected and subsequent measurement of microsphere radioactivity in the collected blood and tissue samples allows microsphere deposition to be converted into blood flow.

Hughes *et al.*[12] examined the blood flow to the intervertebral disk in sheep. Ten adult sheep were injected with approximately 3 million 15 μm microspheres to the left ventricle. Following sacrifice of the animals with an intraventricular injection of saturated potassium chloride, the lumbar spines were removed. At each lumbar disk level, the spines were sectioned to provide two endplate and three disk samples (Figure 3). Each sample was weighed and then counted with the reference sample in a gamma counter.

Regional blood flows were determined using the relationship of sample to reference activity.

$$\text{Blood flow (ml/min/g)} \quad = \quad \frac{\text{Sample activity}}{\text{Reference activity}} \quad x \quad \frac{\text{Withdrawal rate}}{\text{Sample mass}}$$

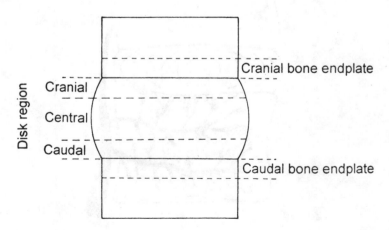

Figure 3. Sections through disc and bone for regional blood flow measurements. (reproduced with permission from Hughes *et al.*, *Europ. Spine J.*, 1993)

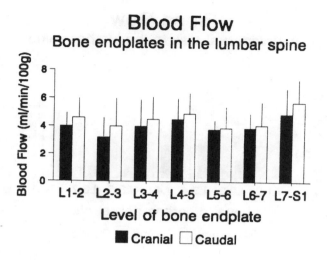

Figure 4. Blood flow in the vertebral endplate at different levels of the ovine lumbar spine. (Reproduced with permission from Hughes *et al.*, *Europ. Spine J.*, 1993)

The vertebral endplates had a mean blood flow of 4.22 ± 0.59 ml/min/100g and there were no significant differences between the different levels of the lumbar spine or between the cranial and caudal endplates at each level. It can be concluded that the blood flow remained constant (Figure 4).

Blood flow to regions of the disk adjoining the endplates were significantly lower and had a mean of 0.57 ± 0.29 ml/min/100g ($P < 0.05$). There were also significant differences between blood flow at the centre of the disk and its extremities (Figure 5). No blood flow could be measured to the nucleus pulposus. Further studies examined the humoral regulation of blood flow in the vertebral endplate and found that the flow was increased by 60% during acetylcholine infusion. This data demonstrates that there are muscarinic receptors in the vessels of the vertebral endplate, which suggests that the vasculature may influence disc nutrition[14].

However, it should not be concluded from the absence of recorded flow in the centre of the disk that there was no blood flow. Microspheres are only entrapped by vessels that are narrower than their 15 μm diameter. If there were to be a blood flow to the nucleus pulposus and the afferent arterioles were smaller than 15 μm, then the microspheres would be trapped before reaching the centre of the disk and no blood flow would be recorded. However, the most likely interpretation of the absence of microspheres in the central region is indeed that there is no blood flow.

There was a clearly evident blood supply to the endplates and to the bone. These values were similar to other measurements made in other bones of other experimental animals. Morris and Kelly[15] observed mean blood flows of 2.46 ml/min/100g in the canine

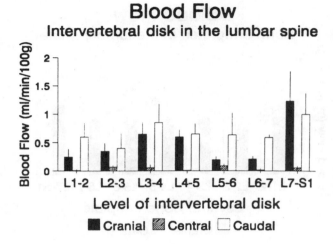

Figure 5. Blood flow in different regions of the intervertebral disc in the ovine lumbar spine. (reproduced with permission from Hughes *et al.*, *Europ. Spine J.*, 1993)

tibial cortex and Strachan *et al.*[16] recorded similar mean blood flows of 3.2 ml/min/100g in the canine tibial cortex. In the sheep, Reichert *et al.*[17] observed that the mean blood flows to the tibial cortex were 0.95 ml/min/100g. These values are all lower than those to the vertebral body.

Physiological measurements of blood flow in the structures of the lumbar spine have been undertaken in humans using positron emission tomography by Ashcroft *et al.*[18] and more recently by Kahn *et al.*[19]. The more recent study used ten normal subjects (5 male, 5 female, age range 20 - 25) shows that the lower lumbar vertebral bodies have a statistically significant higher blood flow (17.6 ml/min/100g, SD = 3.1) than the total superior pelvis (11.1 ml/min/100g, SD = 2.0).

Indirect measurements using magnetic resonance imaging were undertaken by Paajanen *et al.*[20] and were demonstrated to be able to show diurnal fluid changes of lumbar discs. In thirteen healthy subjects the disc signal in T_2-weighted MRI images increased up to 25% after overnight bed rest.

Ahmed *et al.*[21], in an immunohistochemical study using rats, showed that vasoactive neuropeptides such as neuropeptide-Y (NPY), tyrosine hydroxylase (TH) and vasoactive intestinal polypeptide (VIP) are present in the vertebral bodies, annulus fibrosus and spinal ligaments. NPY- and TH-positive nerves, known for their vasoconstrictive properties, were identified in blood vessels in abundance in the cancellous bone and periosteum of the vertebral body as well as the outer layers of the annulus fibrosus. This can be interpreted as an indication of vasoregulatory activity.

4. Clinical Pathology

The importance of the knowledge of the vascular structures around the lumbar spine for the spinal surgeon has been recognized by Crock[22], Anda *et al.*[3] and Smith and Lawrence[24] to avoid intraoperative iatrogenic injury. Postoperative vascular damage and fibrosis within the vertebral canal and intervertebral foramen have been described by Jayson[25] in patients in whom oil-based myelography or spinal surgery was performed.

The role of the vascularity of the lumbar spine in the disease process has not yet been well clarified. Cadaveric studies on non-operated spines showed evidence of vascular damage and fibrosis, seemingly related to the severity of degenerative disc disease[25].

A retrospective study on the coincidence of vertebral bone marrow changes and degenerative lumbar disc disease using MRI undertaken by Toyone *et al.*[26] shows focal bone marrow alterations adjacent to disc degeneration in 94 out of 500 patients. Disc degeneration is shown as decreased signal intensity in the T_2-weighted image. The records of 74 patients with demonstrated vertebral bone marrow changes were complete and examined thoroughly. Two types of bone marrow changes were recognized in the T_1-weighted images. These were designated as types A and B, where type A was observed to exhibit a decreased signal intensity in T_1-weighted images and type B was associated with increased signal intensity in T_1-weighted images. Type A was clearly associated with the clinical picture of severe low back pain, radiological vertebral sclerosis and segmental hypermobility with an anterior-posterior translation exceeding 3 mm. Type B presented with significantly less severe symptoms.

Histological specimens of ten patients grouped type A were available and showed disruption of the endplates, thickened bony trabeculae and fibrovascular bone marrow. Type B histology (5 patients) showed replacement of the marrow with fat. This retrospective study shows disruption of the vertebral endplate and underlying marrow changes in the vertebral body in the presence of degenerative disc disease. It cannot be concluded which of the pathological processes has initiated the degenerative disk disease.

5. Conclusion

Blood flow has been measured in experimental animals and normal subjects in the vertebral body. The importance of the fine structure of the vertebral endplate and its role in the diffusion process of the disc has been recognized. The interrelation between these two structures needs to be evaluated further. The development of imaging techniques will give more insight in the vascularity of the structures of the lumbar spine, although physiological measurements will be difficult. Immunohistochemical staining might allow conclusions about the functional properties of a tissue. Present work in our laboratories is in progress to investigate further the role of the blood supply in lumbar spine disorders.

6. References

1.   J. P. G. Urban, S. Holm, A. Maroudas, *Biorheology* **15** (1978) 203.
2.   H. V. Crock and H. Yoshizawa, *Clin. Orthop.* **115** (1976) 6-21.

3. K. Ogata and L. A. Whiteside, *Spine* **6** (1981) 211-6.
4. J. P. G. Urban, S. Holm, A. Maroudas, A. Nachemson, *Clin. Orthop.* **170** (1982) 296-302.
5. M. Brookes, *The blood supply of bone.* (Butterworths, London, 1971) p. 47.
6. H. V. Crock, M. Goldwasser, H. Yoshizawa, in: *The Biology of the Intervertebral Disc, Vol. 1,* ed. P. Ghosh (CRC Press, Florida, 1988) pp. 109-33.
7. S. Oki, Y. Matsuda, T. Itoh, T. Shibata, H. Okumura, J. Desaki, *J. Orthop. Res.* **12** (1994) 447-9.
8. H. V. Crock, H. Yoshizawa, S. K. Karne, *J. Bone Joint Surg. [Br]* **55-B** (1973) 528-33
9. W. R. Saywell, H. V. Crock, J. P. S. England, R. E. Steiner, *Br. J. Radiol.* **62** (1989) 290-2.
10. H. V. Crock HV, *Acta Orthop. Scand.* **65** (1994) 225-7.
11. G. Breschet, *Recherches anatomiques, physiologiques et pathologiques sur le système veineux, et specialement sur les canaux des os* (Thèse, Paris, 1829).
12. S. P. F. Hughes, A. L. Wallace, I. D. McCarthy, R. H. Fleming, B. C. Wyatt, *Eur Spine J* **2** (1993) 96-8.
13. P. Tothill, *J. Biomed. Eng.* **6** (1984) 251-6.
14. A. L. Wallace, B. C. Wyatt, I. D. McCarthy, S. P. F. Hughes, *Spine* **19** (1994) 1324-8.
15. M. A. Morris and P. J. Kelly, *Calcif. Tissue Int.* **32** (1980) 69-76.
16. R. K. Strachan, I. D. McCarthy, R. Fleming, S. P. F. Hughes, *J. Bone Joint Surg. [Br]* **72-B** (1990) 391-4.
17. I. L. H. Reichert, I. D. McCarthy, S. P. F. Hughes, *J. Bone Joint Surg. [Br]* **in press** (1995).
18. P. Ashcroft, R. W. Porter, N. Evans, D. Roeda, C. Goddard, F. Smith, *J. Bone Joint Surg. [Br]* **74-B Suppl** (1992) 324.
19. D. Kahn, G. J. Weiner, S. Ben-Haim, L. L. Boles Ponto, M. T. Madsen, D. L. Bushnell, G. L. Watkins, E. A. Argenyi, R. D. Hichwa, *Blood* **83** (1994) 958-63.
20. H. Paajanen, I. Lehto, A. Alanen, M. Erkintalo, M. Komu, *J. Orthop. Res.* **12** (1994) 509-14.
21. M. Ahmed, A. Bjurholm, A. Kreicbergs, M. Schultzberg, *Spine* **18** (1993) 268-73.
22. H. V. Crock, *Practice of Spinal Surgery* (Springer Verlag, Wien / New York, 1983).
23. S. Anda, S. Aakhus, K. O. Skaanes, E. Sande, H. Schrader, *Spine* **16** (1991) 54-60.
24. D. W. Smith and B. D. Lawrence, *Spine* **16** (1991) 387-90.
25. M. I. V. Jayson, *Clin. Orthop.* **279** (1992) 40-8.
26. T. Toyone, K. Takahashi, H. Kitahara, M. Yamagata, M. Murakami, H. Moriya, *J. Bone Joint Surg. [Br]* **76-B** (1994) 757-64.

CHAPTER 6

PATHOLOGY OF SYMPTOMATIC LUMBAR DISC PROTRUSION: MEDICO-LEGAL AND SURGICAL IMPLICATIONS

R.W. Porter

1. Introduction

Lower lumbar disc protrusion is the most common spinal condition treated by surgeons, who need to keep abreast of the major advances in understanding its pathophysiology. New concepts on the function of the disc in health and disease, and the significance of the abnormal signs, have important therapeutic and medico-legal implications, and there is a danger that new imaging techniques might outpace surgeons' clinical skills.

2. Physiology

2.1. Morphology

The remarkable structure of the intervertebral disc makes the spine both supple and strong. When subjected to axial loads, the disc is stronger than the vertebrae. Bone will fracture before the disc fails. The radial-ply design of the annulus is responsible for its strength. Each layer has parallel fibres at approximately 30 degrees to the horizontal, but in the opposite direction to the adjacent layer. When the disc is loaded the laminated collagen is in tension, and the annulus merely bulges. The large molecules of proteoglycan in the nucleus attract water, achieving a balance with the spine's hydrostatic pressure. In health this is a very strong system.

However, the collagen fibres fail in more than three degrees of disc torsion[1]. One layer of the annulus will deform beyond its elastic limit. This is normally restrained by the sagittal orientation of the apophyseal joints, and by the splinting effects of the spinal muscles and the intra-abdominal pressure.

2.2. Nutrition

The disc is the largest avascular structure in the body. The cells in the disc turn over collagen and proteoglycan, and must receive nutrients and eliminate metabolites. They require an efficient diffusion pathway[2]. It is through the vertebral endplate that diffusion largely occurs, and its blood supply is therefore critical.

Passive diffusion depends on a balance between the osmotic and hydrostatic pressure of the disc. During recumbency, with a reduced hydrostatic load, fluid is imbibed by the discs, resulting in 17 mm diurnal change in stature. This will benefit small molecular diffusion, and thus a post-prandial slumber may keep the discs healthy!

However, there may also be an active component to disc nutrition. The vessels supplying the end-plate are terminal branches of the lumbar arteries and they have an unusual structure. Many are tortuous, resembling the glomerular vessels, and are probably under autonomic control[3]. Acetylcholine produces a significant increase in end-plate blood flow, suggesting the presence of muscarine receptors in the vascular bed[4]. Nicotine may also have a potent effect on end-plate blood flow. Studies of identical twins, only one of whom smokes, have shown significant reduction in disc hydration in the smoking twin[5]. Smoking is also known to be a risk factor for back pain. There is also a high incidence of back pain in occupations subject to vibration[6-8], which may also affect endplate circulation and disc nutrition.

Disc failure and pathological change may therefore result more from impairment of disc nutrition than from mechanical causes.

3. Pathology

3.1. Mechanical stress

Disc nutrition cannot be the whole explanation of disc failure, otherwise one would expect all the lumbar discs to be equally affected by pathological change. MRI studies, however, frequently show one or two degenerate discs, while adjacent discs are well hydrated. It is probable that poor nutrition makes a disc vulnerable to damage by either peak loads or repetitive minor loads. The disc begins to fissure, and once damaged, because of the low metabolic rate, repair is unlikely to keep pace with further pathological change[2]. Fissures progress throughout the nucleus to the periphery of the annulus. Of clinical significance is the double fissure, which produces a 'doughnut' appearance, with the formation of a loose fragment.

3.2. Disc protrusion

It is difficult in the laboratory to produce a protrusion by applying an axial load to an isolated spine. Enormous loads in non-physiological hyperflexion can rupture a healthy disc, but this probably does not occur in life. Even if a fissure is artificially created in a disc, it is not possible to produce a protrusion by loading the segment. However, if a fragment of disc material from another disc is introduced into that fissure, it takes only minimal physiological loads (1 kN) to produce a protrusion[9]. The posterior annulus will bulge and sometimes rupture as the free fragment is extruded, much like a pea squeezed out of a pod. If the laboratory situation is true to life, it is probable that a disc protrusion cannot occur unless there is both a disc fissure and also a free or almost-free fragment. Once the fragment has formed, it does not take much of a load to cause a protrusion, or even a complete rupture of the annulus.

3.3. Medico-legal implications of the 'fissure and fragment'

Many patients with symptomatic disc protrusion can recollect an acute onset to their first symptoms—more than patients with other back pain syndromes[10]. They remember an incident when they twisted or bent forwards, perhaps carrying a load, which they describe as an 'injury'. The first pain can be agonizing. It is imprinted on the memory, and if it occurred at work is thought worthy of compensation. However, the first symptom is merely the end-result of a long-standing symptomless process, which would inevitably have occurred whenever the spine was subject to this degree of load. Even lesser repetitive loads could cause the protrusion. Thus when the first symptoms occur when lifting, twisting or bending they are an incident in a long-standing process, and not an accident. It would probably not have been long before a similar load produced a similar problem.

3.4. Surgical implications of the 'fissure and fragment'

Surgeons have been unsure whether it is necessary to remove a large amount of disc material, or whether simple excision of the fragment will suffice. If it is correct that a degenerate disc with a fissure does not cause protrusion, but rather the loose fragment is responsible for symptoms, then it is reasonable to remove only the fragment at surgery. It is probably good practice to explore cautiously for semi-loose fragments that may subsequently separate and cause trouble, but radical removal of a large quantity of annulus is now unnecessary.

3.5. The vertebral canal

The size and shape of the vertebral canal are critical in the development of symptoms from a disc protrusion. If the vertebral canal is sufficiently wide, the nerve roots of the cauda equina are spared from compression. The posterior annulus is stretched, causing back pain and/or referred pain, but there is no root pain. However, if the vertebral canal is shallow in the sagittal plane, or trefoil in shape, the nerve root is rapidly compromised. Fifty per cent of patients whose symptomatic disc protrusion causes sciatic pain have vertebral canals in the bottom tenth percentile of the normal population[11]. Patients with wider canals may have disc protrusion, but they escape disabling root symptoms. By 60 years of age, one-third of the population has sustained a disc protrusion, but most are symptomless[12]. This is because most of them are fortunate enough to have a wide vertebral canal.

3.6. Inflammation

Disc protrusion with mechanical compression of the nerve root does not explain the whole mechanism of root symptoms. Nerve roots are frequently compressed by degenerative bone, capsule, or ligamentum flavum, without developing root-tension signs. Similarly, root-tension signs vary with time in spite of a constant protrusion size on imaging. Furthermore, straight leg raising recovers only slowly after surgical removal of a disc protrusion, even though the compression is relieved. The phenomenon of the root-tension sign can best be explained by an inflammatory process mediated by the nucleus pulposus on a compressed root.

In a pig model, nucleus pulposus has a profound effect on the cauda equina, inducing chemotactic signals that attract inflammatory cells[13-14]. It is probable that these inflammatory changes are responsible for the acute root symptoms, and for the root oedema frequently seen on MRI for many months after a successful discectomy. Figure 1 summarises the pathological process responsible for symptomatic disc protrusion.

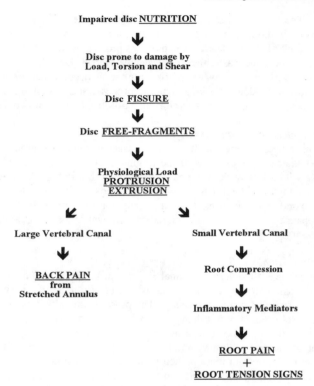

Figure 1. Pathological process of symptomatic disc protrusion.

4. Symptomatology

4.1. Trunk list

The only objective sign that is pathognomonic of disc protrusion is a trunk list. Other signs can be influenced by subjectivity, but the trunk list is beyond the patient's control. Its mechanism is unknown. It is present in about 50% of patients with a protrusion. It is gravity induced, being abolished when the patient lies down or hangs from a bar. Twice as many patients list to the left than to the right. It is unrelated to the side of the sciatica, to the level or the side of the lesion, and it is unrelated to the topographical position of the disc—axillary, anterior or lateral[15]. It carries a poor prognosis for conservative management, about 30% of these patients requiring surgery[16].

4.2. Straight leg raising

Straight leg raising is the important pathognomonic root-tension sign of disc protrusion. The exaggerating patient can be detected by internally rotating the extended leg, which normally increases the pain, and externally rotating the leg, which relieves the pain[17]. The flip test extends the knee of the seated patient, who should flip over backwards if the root tension sign is genuine. Cross leg pain, when pain is experienced in the symptomatic leg when raising the other leg, also carries a poor prognosis for conservative care; 50% of these patients will ultimately require surgery[16].

Bladder dysfunction is the only absolute indication for early surgery in a patient with disc protrusion. Surgery is unnecessary when straight leg raising is better than 50 degrees, provided the patient is prepared to wait for recovery. These patients ultimately do as well treated conservatively as by operation[18]. However, many are impatient and early expeditious surgery will relieve the root pain. Risks are remote but significant.

4.3. Imaging

Only when the decision to operate has been made is imaging requested, not to diagnose the condition but to identify its level. The choice of imaging depends on resources, but MRI is the method of choice. Using imaging as a 'fishing trip' to make a diagnosis is poor practice. It is likely to confuse the issue and reveal protrusions that may be clinically irrelevant[19]. However, we can now anticipate excellent results with improved assessment, precise imaging and expeditious surgery.

5. References

1. D.S. Hickey and D.W.L. Hukins, *Spine* **5** (1980) 106.
2. J. Urban, in *The Lumbar Spine*, eds. J.N. Weinstein and S.W. Wiesel (W.B. Saunders, San Francisco, 1990) p. 231.
3. R.W. Porter, *Management of Back Pain*, 2nd edn. (Churchill Livingstone, Edinburgh, 1994) p. 53.
4. S.P.F. Hughes, A.L. Wallace, I.D. McCarthy, R.H. Fleming and B.C. Wyatt, The regulation of blood flow in the vertebral end plate. Presented to the International Society for the Study of the Lumbar Spine, Marseilles, 1993.
5. M.C.M. Battie, T. Videman and K. Gill, *Spine* **9** 1991 164.
6. J.A.D. Anderson, *J. Soc. Occup. Med.* **36** (1986) 90.
7. H.C. Boshinzen, P.M. Bongers and C.T.J. Hulshof, *Spine* **17** (1992) 59.
8. J.G. Fitzgerald and J. Crotty, The incidence of backache among air crew and ground crew in the Royal Air Force. Flying Personnel Research Committee—Ministry of Defence (Air Force Department) 1972; FPRC/1313.
9. P. Brinkman and R.W. Porter, *Spine* **19** (1994) 228.
10. K.M.K. Varma, *Sudden onset back pain*. Thesis, University of Liverpool, 1990.
11. R.W. Porter, M. Wicks and C. Hibbert, *J. Bone Joint Surg.* **60-B** (1978) 485.
12. S.D. Boden, D.O. Davis, T.S. Dina, N.J. Patronas and S.W. Weisel, *J Bone Joint Surg.* **72-A** (1990) 403.
13. M. Cornefjord, K. Olmarker, D.B. Farley, J.N. Weinstein and B. Rydevik, Substance P and VIP in spinal nerve roots after epidural application of autologous nucleus pulposus. *Neuro-Orthopaedics*, in press 1996.

14.   M. Doita, T. Kanatani, T. Harada and K. Mizuno, *Spine* **20** (1996) 2613.
15.   R.W. Porter and C. Miller, *Spine* **11** (1986) 596.
16.   B. Khuffash, R.W. Porter, *Spine* **14** (1989) 602.
17.   A. Breig and J.D.G. Troup, *Spine* **4** (1979) 242.
18.   H. Weber, *Spine* **8** (1983) 131.
19.   N. Boos, R. Rieder, V. Schade, K.F. Spratt, N. Semmer and M. Aebi, *Spine* **20** (1995) 2613.

CHAPTER 7

MAGNETIC RESONANCE IMAGING
OF THE LUMBAR SPINE

P. Thorpe and F.W. Smith

1. Introduction

It has long been recognised that radiographic signs of degeneration seen on plain lumbar spine films bear little relation to clinical symptoms. Myelography extended the realm of imaging to the thecal sac and ultimately, with water soluble contrast media, to the nerve roots themselves. This however is an invasive procedure, and is only diagnostically useful if cerebro-spinal fluid displacement has occurred, giving no direct indication as to the cause of this displacement. Computerised tomography provided the first global picture of the canal and its contents but is constrained by very limited soft tissue contrast, single plane imaging and the high radiation burden entailed in the examination of multiple levels. Magnetic resonance overcomes these disadvantages, offering excellent and variable soft tissue contrast, not purely dependent on small differences in X-ray attenuation. The ability to image in multiple planes greatly aids an overall appreciation of the significance of abnormal findings as well as serving to screen the spine, often demonstrating pathology at the levels remote from those suspected clinically. The technique uses no ionising radiation and is without known side effects. Magnetic resonance imaging (MRI) constitutes the most important single advance in methods for investigating the lumbar spine. For the first time the power of the tool is ahead of our understanding of pathology, an important caveat for interpreting images and the reason why the technique poses at least as many questions as it answers.

Contrast in a magnetic resonance image is dependent on the physical environment of hydrogen atoms and their nuclei in the tissues being imaged. Hydrogen nuclei may be thought of as being like spinning bar magnets. When they are placed in a magnetic field, the axis of the magnet starts to turn, or precess, about the direction of that field, like a child's spinning top wobbling about its axis. The frequency of precession (how fast it turns) depends on the strength of the magnetic field. There is, therefore, a characteristic frequency associated with each hydrogen nucleus in a given magnetic field. Nuclear magnetic resonance occurs because the nuclei can absorb electromagnetic energy at this characteristic frequency, which turns out to be at about the frequency of radio waves. A simple mechanical analogy is a child on a swing[2]. Pushing at the right frequency, *i.e.* every time the swing passes will then make the child swing higher. Pushing at any other frequency will have little effect and may even hinder the motion of the swing. Returning to the hydrogen nuclei in the body, they can be given energy by a pulse of radio-waves at the right frequency. When the radio frequency pulse is discontinued, the nuclei lose the extra energy and return to their resting state in the magnetic field, a process called 'relaxation'. This energy that they give up is again at radio-frequencies and can be collected by receiving coils placed around the patient. It is from these signals that the image is calculated.

Much of the soft tissue of the body has a similar water content (70 - 80%) so that an image made up merely from the density of hydrogen nuclei at a given location would have poor contrast. Fortunately, the rate at which hydrogen nuclei lose energy is influenced by their surroundings. This environment varies between tissues and is markedly different in many disease states, especially neoplasia. It is primarily this environmental influence on nuclear relaxation that imparts tissue contrast to an MR image. There are principally two different ways in which the nuclei can give up their energy; both to the atoms of the surrounding molecules (often called the lattice because all the early NMR work was done on crystalline materials which have a lattice structure) and to adjacent spinning nuclei. A measure of the time taken for a given nucleus to give up its energy by either one of these mechanisms is called the relaxation time. So, energy loss to the surroundings is chracterised by T1, or the spin-lattice, relaxation time and that to adjacent nuclei by the T2, or spin-spin, relaxation time. The parameters employed to collect the image can be adjusted so that either one of these relaxation types predominate in the final image (although the effect of the other can never be totally eliminated). Each given tissue will have certain values for T1 and T2 relaxation times and these will generate contrast in T1- and T2-weighted images. Cerebro-spinal fluid (CSF), for example, has a high unbound water content and will return a high signal on T2 images (bright) and low signal on T1 images (dark). In contrast, fat returns a high signal on both (Table 1).

Table 1. Description of the appearance of various tissues in a spin-echo image

	Low signal (dark)				High signal (bright)	
	Long T1					Short T1
T1-weighted image	Air Cortical bone	Water	White matter	Grey matter Muscle Spleen	Liver	Fat
	Short T2					Long T2
T2-weighted image	Air Cortical bone		Liver	Muscle White matter	Kidney Spleen Grey matter	Water Fat

Producing T1 and T2 images is done not by using just one radio-frequency pulse as described above but by using a series of pulses of carefully defined lengths and intervals that selectively enable one or the other relaxation time to be recorded. This is called a pulse sequence. Perhaps the most common is the spin-echo sequence but many others have been developed in an attempt to decrease image acquisition times and increase tissue discrimination. These go under such exotic names as turbo spin-echo, gradient echo or inversion recovery sequences (STIR- short-tau inversion recovery) for instance. All of these sequences will influence tissue contrast and signal parameters in different ways and need care and experience for their interpretation.

2. The standard lumbar spine examination

The standard lumbar spine examination is performed with the patient relaxed, lying supine on a dedicated lumbar spine receive coil. It should commence with a T2-weighted sagittal sequence which exploits the unique ability of MR to examine the lumbar spine in its entirety. Many patients have pathology at levels other than those clinically suspected. Prolapsed disc material is easily recognised on these T2 images by indentation of the high signal of the CSF sac (Figure 1) or displacement of perineural fat in the exit foramen on the parasagittal images (Figure 2). Although sensitive to disc pathology, the degree of disc prolapse may be exaggerated on T2 images. Corroboration of suspected prolapse by T1 images in the sagittal or axial planes is thus essential. The relationship between extruded disc material and the posterior longitudinal ligament (PLL) is apparent on the sagittal images. This relationship is important to the surgeon as a prolapse completely contained by the PLL may be difficult to appreciate operatively. The parasagittal images give a good impression of the degree of nerve root encroachment by a posterolateral disc (Figure 2) and should be carefully studied, again relating any findings to the axial images. Extreme lateral or anterior disc prolapses are best appreciated on axial images. Extension of a central prolapse beneath the PLL is readily seen and the sequestered fragment is the undoubted forté of a sagittal sequence (Figure 3). No other imaging modality demonstrates the sequestrum and its relationship to the parent disc so elegantly.

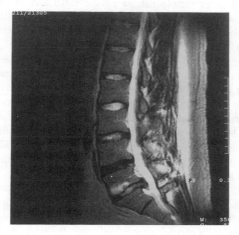

Figure 1. A T2 weighted sagittal image showing a posterior disc prolapse at the lumbo-sacral junction. Note the elevation of the posterior longitudinal ligament and the pronounced endplate change in the lower margin of L5. This was a type 2 endplate change as there was a corresponding area of high signal on the T1 weighted sequence.

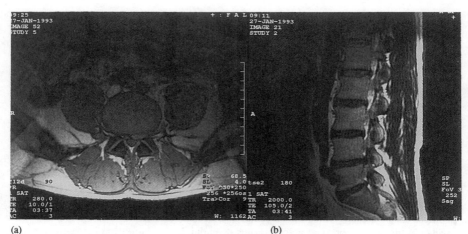

(a)   (b)

Figure 2. An axial image (a) confirms that disc material is obliterating the axilla of the exit foramen at L4/5 and L5/S1 as shown by the T2 parasagittal sequence (b).

T1-weighted axial images are made through discs at levels suspected clinically and those demonstrating abnormality on the T2 sequence. The default examination would acquire images from the lowermost three levels as discs here account for the majority of symptomatic disc protrusions. The T1 sequence gives a further perspective on the degree of foraminal impingement and confirms the radiological significance of the abnormalities seen on the T2 study. It provides the most accurate anatomical localisation of the prolapse and an appreciation of other factors narrowing the canal and therefore increasing the significance of prolapsed nuclear material. Thus spinal stenosis from flaval hypertrophy or abnormal canal morphology as well as narrowing of the lateral recess is readily appreciated (Figure 4).

Short Tau Inversion Recovery (STIR) images in the coronal plane are a useful adjunct to basic, fast spin echo sequences. This study provides an automyelogram using the patients own CSF as contrast (Figure 5). It serves both to confirm thecal compression from equivocal discs and to demonstrate CSF surrounding the nerve roots in a second plane (Figure 6). Spinal stenosis is beautifully demonstrated by the STIR sequence (Figure 7). The most significant levels are most easily determined by this study which is directly comparable to the standard myelogram in these circumstances. 3D rendering further produces visually pleasing images but rarely provides additional information in the lumbar spine although its use in the cervical spine is now well established.

If appropriate pathology is demonstrated by the above sequences the examination is terminated at this point. Total imaging time with modern, fast scanning protocols is about 15 minutes (Table 2). If the above sequences are normal then a T2-weighted whole spine image to include the medulla should be acquired using the body receiver coil to exclude proximal pathology (Figure 8).

The vertebral bodies should be examined at this point. On both T1- and T2-weighted

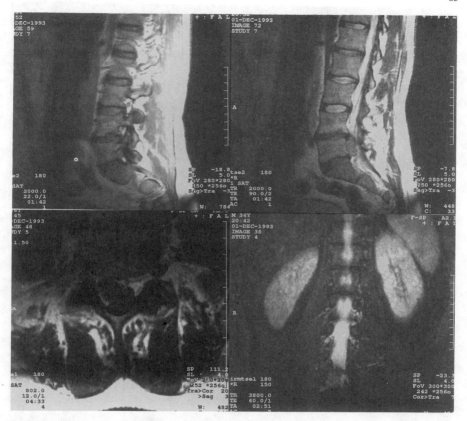

Figure 3. (Top left) A large sequestered disc is demonstrated by the sagittal T2 sequence to descend behind the vertebral body of L5. The parasagittal (top right) and axial (bottom left) images show impingement on the right exit foramen. The S.T.I.R. sequence (bottom right) elegantly demonstrates the filling defect in the CSF

sequences, cortical bone appears black due to the relative lack of hydrogen nuclei whilst medullary bone is grey. The remnant of the developmental cleft is often seen in the posterior aspect of the vertebral body as a light grey line.

Three types of change in the vertebral body end plates have been described[3]. In acute degenerative disc disease there is often an associated inflammatory reaction in the endplates which appears dark on T1- and white on T2-weighted images (Type I). These changes are seen in patients with active degeneration or instability and correlate well with the patient's symptoms. Subsequent fatty infiltration, appearing white on T1- and grey on T2-weighted images characterise Type II changes and imply established degeneration. Type III changes reflect sub-endplate sclerosis with loss of signal on both sequences and represent end stage disease.

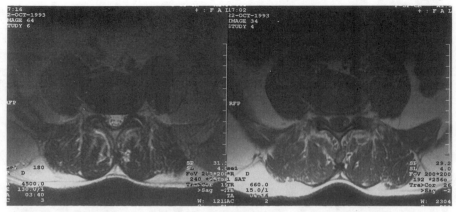

Figure 4. T2 and T1 axial images demonstrating stenosis of the left nerve root exit foramen by soft tissue hypertrophy associated with the facet joint. Under these circumstances even a small disc bulge will be significant.

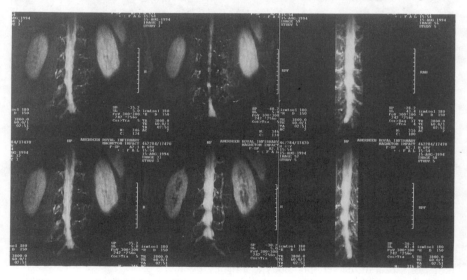

Figure 5. A normal coronal STIR sequence re-registered as a maximum intensity projection (M.I.P.) allowing viewing from multiple angles analogous to oblique views in conventional contrast myelography.

The presence of areas of high signal on the T2 images within the vertebral bodies requires a T1 sequence to characterise the abnormality. The most common cause will be vertebral haemangiomata which also appear white on T1 (Figure 9). High T2 and low T1 signal is less specific, merely suggesting a higher unbound water content than surrounding

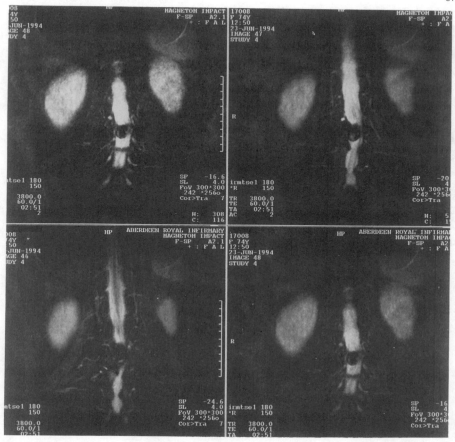

Figure 6. Coronal STIR images demonstrating the CSF filling defect produced by a posterior disc prolapse.

bone, thus both benign lesions *e.g.* Schmorl's nodes, and malignant lesions, *e.g.* metastases (Figure 10) would give this appearance. Diagnosis is usually possible from the location and distribution of the abnormality and a knowledge of the clinical circumstances. Having completed the examination, comment can be made on vertebral integrity and alignment, the size and nature of disc pathology, the presence and cause of spinal stenosis, posterior degenerative change and the condition of the paraspinal soft tissues throughout the lumbar spine. Although much of this information can be shown or inferred from conventional investigations, no other modality is able to demonstrate all of these structures in one study and thus provide an overall view of the pathological anatomy of the low back.

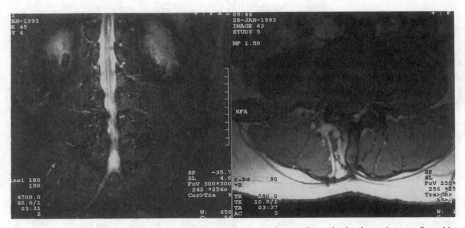

Figure 7. The coronal STIR sequence demonstrates spinal stenosis over the entire lumbar spine, confirmed by axial sections.

Table 2. A standard series of sequences for lumbar spine imaging at 1 Tesla

Sequence	T1	T2	T2	STIR
Orientation	Sagittal	Sagittal	Axial	Coronal
Time to repetition (ms)	600	4500	4400	2500
Time to inversion (ms)	-	-	-	150
Time to echo (ms)	12	130	128	60
Acquisition time (min:sec)	3:04	2:45	4:07	1:52
Slice thickness (mm)	4	4	4	5
Field of view	300	280	128	300
Matrix	240x256	252x256	368x512	242x250

3. Intervertebral disc disease

The resolution, soft tissue contrast and multi-planar capabilities of MRI make an anatomical description of the site of disc pathology relatively easy. Interpretation of the significance of any abnormality demonstrated is more difficult and cannot be the province of the radiologist in isolation. MR abnormalities must be placed within the context of a preceding thorough clinical assessment and the interpretation of images should ideally occur in the surroundings of a clinico-radiological conference.

The structure of a normal intervertebral disc is best demonstrated on T2-weighted

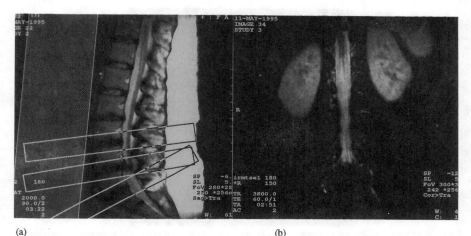

(a)   (b)

Figure 8. Multiple pathology. The distal thoracic meningioma is shown on the scout view (a) but is better demonstrated by the STIR (b).

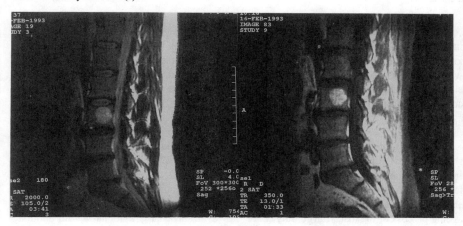

Figure 9. T1 and T2 weighted sagittal sequences showing the typical high signal of a vertebral haemangioma.

images (Figure 11). The relatively high unbound water content of the nucleus pulposus returns a high signal. In the mature skeleton this signal surrounds the central low signal intranuclear cleft, orientated parallel to the endplate. This is the same structure evident on the normal discogram (Figure 12). It is not evident on gross inspection of the nucleus but corresponds to a local reduction in proteoglycan concentration seen on histological sections[1]. Development of the intranuclear cleft reflects maturation of the disc and further ageing of the nucleus is reflected on T2 images by the gradual loss of signal indicating nuclear desiccation.

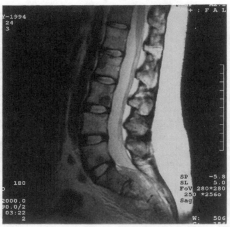

Figure 10. Multiple spinal metastases from malignant melanoma T2 sagittal study. The paramagnetic properties of melanin decrease signal on T2 images in distinction to the high signal more usually seen in other metastatic deposits.

The annulus returns homogeneously low signal. High signal within the annular region implies the presence of free water or nuclear material, *i.e.* a tear. As in the menisci of the knee, tears may be degenerative or traumatic in origin and the orientation of the fluid within the annulus may be important. It has been suggested that tears extending circumferentially through the fibres of the annulus are more likely to be degenerative and are of less significance than radially orientated tears. Radial tears are common in younger age groups, may themselves be a cause of discogenic pain and may predispose to nuclear extrusion.

There is some confusion regarding the terminology of annular degeneration. A 'bulge' should suggest degenerative laxity of the annulus fibrosis which combined with a change in nuclear viscosity, again degenerative in origin, allows indentation of the posterior longitudinal ligament and thecal sac beyond the posterior longitudinal vertebral lines. The significance of a disc bulge is uncertain, as again the phenomenon forms part of the normal ageing process of the disc. Large bulges are, however, invariably associated with annular tears and are likely to be symptomatic or to progress to protrusion. Signal within the annulus in association with the bulge therefore raises the significance of this finding[7]. A discogram may still be required to determine the significance of a disc bulge, as tears are more convincingly demonstrated and stress testing of the disc during the investigation still remains the gold standard for determining the presence of discogenic pain.

Nuclear protrusion implies a more localised area of annular degeneration or defect. Nuclear material may be contained by a few annular fibres or there may be frank nuclear extrusion. The differentiation between protrusion and extrusion is academic as extruded nuclear material produces a fibrous response which contains the extrusion in the majority of cases. Protrusions may be central, postero-lateral (the most common site), lateral, extreme lateral or anterior with distinct clinical symptoms attributable to each of these

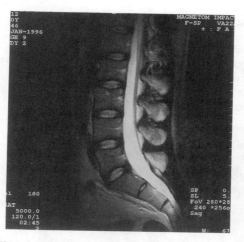

Figure 11. Normal T2 sagittal study to show the morphology of normal young intervertebral discs. The well hydrated nucleus outlines the low signal of the intranuclear cleft. Compare this appearance to that seen on the normal discogram (Figure 12).

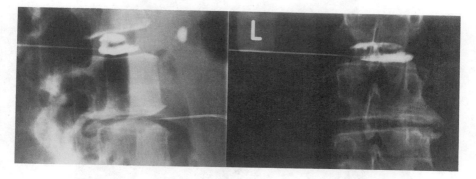

Figure 12. A normal discogram demonstrating the intervertebral cleft.

locations. Thus a postero-lateral protrusion commonly compromises the nerve root exiting below the degenerate level (a L4/5 postero-lateral protrusion producing L5 symptoms). A lateral or extreme lateral protrusion however would be expected to give symptoms or signs relating to the same dermatomal level. Overlap and blurring of clinical symptoms is, however, common. Sequestration occurs when disc material separates from its parent disc and migrates along the canal producing very variable clinical signs. MR is the modality of choice to demonstrate this phenomenon.

4. Pathology mimicking disc disease

Soft tissue filling the exit foramen from any cause will mimic disc protrusion. This may be a normal anatomical variant such as a conjoint nerve root (Figure 13). Arachnoid or Tarlov cysts of the nerve roots will appear as soft tissue density on CT and can give rise to confusion. These structures would share the characteristics of CSF on all MR sequences and errors should not therefore occur (Figure 14).

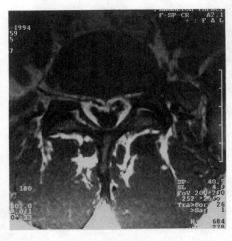

Figure 13. Asymmetry in the size of the nerve roots on this axial image is due to a conjoined root on the left. When adjacent to the posterior aspect of the disc this appearance can be misinterpreted as impinging disc material.

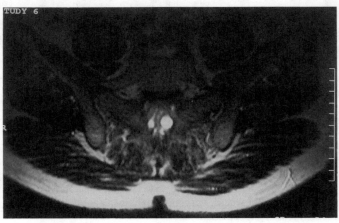

Figure 14. Sacral T2 axial oblique image to show the high (CSF) signal of bilateral Tarlov cysts.

Early case reports described spontaneous resolution of disc protrusions. Whilst this is seen over a period of some months in clinical practice undoubtedly some reports outlining rapidly resolving protrusions were describing extradural haematomata. The appearance of blood on MR images varies with the age of the collection and the sequence used (Table 3). Haematomata originating from the point of entry of the vertebro-basillar veins into the vertebral body will be centred at the mid-point of the vertebral body as opposed to disc level. Although the site of the abnormality can be useful in differentiating haematoma from a protruded disc, differentiation from a sequestered fragment in the presence of degenerate discs is difficult. The correct diagnosis will depend on a high clinical suspicion and repeat studies.

Table 3. variation from an evolving haematoma at 1.5 Tesla

Age of haematoma	T1 Signal	T2 Signal	Predominant haemoglobin molecule
0 - 6 hours	N/↓	↑	Oxyhaemoglobin
6 hours - Days	N/↑	↓	Deoxyhaemoglobin
Days - Week	↑↑	↓↓	Intracellular methaemoglobin
Week - Months	↑↑	↑↑	Extracellular methaemoglobin
Chronic	↓	↓↓	Haemosiderin

The distinction between recurrent disc and scar tissue in the post-operative spine is of paramount importance. Further surgery on the spinal canal that has already demonstrated a propensity towards exuberant scarring is clearly undesirable. A contrast-enhanced MR is now the method of choice in differentiating scar tissue from recurrent disc material and enables an accurate diagnosis in 96% of cases[6]. By comparison, CT has an accuracy accepted at 70 to 80%, comparable with that of an unenhanced MR.

Images should be made within a few minutes of contrast administration. In this period increased signal will be due to contrast within the vascular or immediate peri-vascular space owing to the imperfect intracellular junctions of new vessels within granulation scar tissue. After 30 minutes contrast may have redistributed so that enhancement less reliably reflects vascularity. Images made at this stage may show enhancement of herniated disc material. Examined in this way, contrast enhancement is a reliable differentiator of scar and disc material many years after an operative procedure. Misinterpretation is possible when scar tissue surrounds or invades disc material. Rim enhancement is often a feature of established herniations and must be differentiated from the more homogeneous enhancement expected within scar tissue. Further differentiating evidence may be the position of the mass, its shape within the canal, the presence of mass effect and its continuity with adjacent disc material. All of these features however show some overlap and are probably best used to support the impression gained by the behaviour of the mass following Gadolinium administration. All of the above caveats also apply to contrast enhanced CT.

Apart from in the post-operative spine, the use of intravenous contrast during a routine MR lumbar spine examination is not in widespread use and is probably not cost effective. A small study of 30 patients showed an increase in confidence at only 1 in 10 lumbar levels examined[5]. Intravenous contrast in these circumstances rarely shows an abnormality not appreciated on unenhanced images although significantly compressed nerve roots do enhance. It may however be of use to characterise or improve the anatomical definition of lesions such as meningioma (Figure 15) or neurofibroma. Intrathecal contrast has no place in MR evaluation. The high unbound water in CSF can provide all the contrast necessary for an auto-myelogram when T2 weighted or STIR sequences are employed (Figure 5).

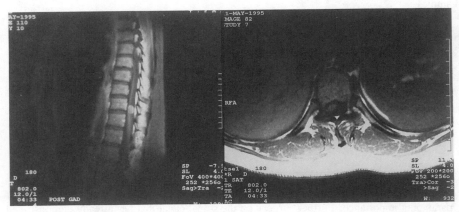

Figure 15. Contrast enhancement is useful to define the extent of spinal tumours and their relationship to the cord as with this meningioma (unenhanced T1 axial, enhanced T1 sagittal).

5. Lumbar spine tumours

The most common tumour of the lumbar spine is the vertebral haemangioma. This neoplasm is seen in 10-20% of routine lumbar MR examinations and is more common than plain film radiographs would suggest. Its appearances on MR are characteristic. The relatively high fat content of the tumour, together with the presence of slow flowing blood, give high signal on both T1 and T2 studies. These appearances are virtually pathognomonic. Occasionally, examples are seen with multiple haemangiomata spread throughout the lumbar spine. Metastases, however, would be expected to return high signal on T2 studies and low signal on T1. Melanoma metastases are an exception and characteristically appear white on T1 and dark on T2 images due to the presence of paramagnetic melanin. The differentiation between metastatic deposits and herniation of disc material through an osteoporotic endplate can occasionally be difficult, although other signs of osteoporosis, the proximity of all lesions to endplates and continuity of signal across the endplate usually help. True Schmorl's nodes seen in the younger population are generally multiple and more evident in the thoracic than the lumbar spine.

The presence of neurofibromata may be suspected from the plain film appearances of pedicular narrowing and foraminal widening. Again, their MR appearances tend to be characteristic with high signal on T2 images, signal isointense with cord on T1 and avid contrast enhancement. Nerve roots can also be expanded by the formation of arachnoid cysts or Tarlov cysts of the nerve root sheaths. These are often multiple and, as would be expected, have the characteristics of unbound water on MR (Figure 14). Apparent thickening of the nerve roots may also be caused by two roots exiting at the same level so called conjoined root (Figure 13). This fusiform swelling of the nerve root within the exit foramen is more commonly confused with extruded disc material than tumour. The differentiation lies in following the fate of the thickened nerve root over multiple axial sections.

Myeloma may also cause extensive vertebral body destruction indistinguishable on MR from metastatic disease. Myeloma is said to affect the vertebral body whereas metastases affect primarily the pedicles and posterior elements. This rule is too much of a generalisation to be of practical use. In practice, the haematological manifestations of myelogram will enable a diagnosis to be made. If these are unhelpful, bone biopsy is usually necessary.

Other spinal tumours are rare by comparison and would even more rarely present by mimicking disc disease. There are two points that should be made concerning intra- and extra-axial tumours in routine lumbar spine scanning. Firstly, the use of Gadolinium in day-to-day lumbar spine work is not justified as the numbers of tumours encountered is small and Gadolinium does not increase sensitivity. However, if a suspect lesion is encountered it is imperative to acquire both T1 and T2 images and if the characteristics of haemangioma are not demonstrated then Gadolinium enhancement will help to characterise further the extent and nature of the lesion. Secondly, if no cause for the patient's symptoms is demonstrated by the routine lumbar spine sequences described above, T2 sagittal whole spine images should be acquired to exclude a cephalad lesion. This extra sequence will have a low sensitivity but the added peace of mind that it imparts is worth an extra 3 minutes in the magnet.

6. Spondylolisthesis

Axial imaging of spondylolisthesis presents problems due to the finite thickness of the cartilage and partial volume average of bone, disc and theca. The sagittal and coronal planes available from a standard MR study facilitate interpretation of the axial images and are essential in establishing the integrity of the disc involved. Vertebral morphology is also demonstrated by the sagittal images and the lytic defect itself can be demonstrated with appropriate orientation of the scanning plane. The lytic defect may not be evident on axial CT sections unless a reverse gantry angle is used.

7. Arachnoiditis

The appearance of the cauda equina within the lumbar tissues can be very variable. The normal spine may demonstrate peripheral conglomerations of nerve roots, especially at upper lumbar levels. Conjoined nerve roots may also be interpreted erroneously as pathologically adherent roots. Clumping of nerve roots distally is more likely to be pathological. Ross *et al.*[4] described three appearances dependent on whether the nerve roots were clumped centrally, peripherally or diffusely in the thecal sac, sometimes almost totally obliterating the subarachnoid space. These appearances should suggest diagnosis when seen in the clinical scenario of continued back pain following spinal surgery or injection. MR appearances correlate with CT and myelography.

8. Contraindications to MR scanning

No long term deleterious effects of the magnetic field or the radio frequency energy involved in MR imaging have been demonstrated. The strong magnetic field can interfere with electronic devices such as pacemakers, implantable stimulators and syringe pumps. Ferro-magnetic material can also undergo movement as the patient moves across the magnetic field. For this reason patients with metallic foreign bodies adjacent to the eye and recently applied steel aneurysm clips should not be imaged. However, subcutaneous foreign bodies which may not be recognised by the patient may still cause pain because of this movement. When located within the imaged field these foreign bodies produce local signal void and may produce more generalised field inhomogeneity and distortion. The magnitude of this artefact will depend more on the paramagnetic properties of the foreign body rather than its size. Thus small segments of drill bit or scalpel blade remaining following surgery may cause relatively more distortion than large fusion plates (Figure 16).

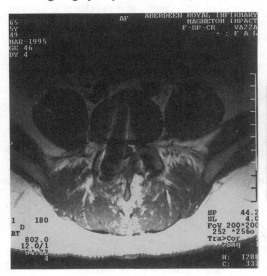
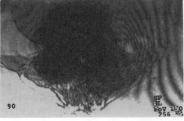

Figure 16. Right, a T1 axial image showing the marked signal drop out and distortion caused by stainless steel pedicular screws. Despite the larger volume of metal, the distortion caused by titanium Steffi plate screws is less noticeable (left), allowing diagnostic images to be acquired.

Metallic fragments or dust in the patient's clothing which transfer to the bore of the magnet or imaging table can markedly reduce image quality and are very difficult to remove, for this reason patients should always be imaged in a hospital gown. The most common limiting factor in MR imaging is claustrophobia and approximately 2% of patients will not tolerate the close confines of the magnet bore. Rapidly changing electrical currents produce an appreciable amount of noise which is especially disturbing to young patients. This can be masked by negative noise or more simply by ear plugs.

The lack of ionising radiation, compared with X-ray examination, makes MRI especially suitable for the young population afflicted by back pain. A CT scan of the lumbar spine at 3 levels is equivalent to approximately 200 chest X-rays. Women are still not imaged in the first trimester of pregnancy unless there is clinical urgency although this has never been proven to be harmful to the foetus.

The advantages of MRI are its ability to demonstrate both bone and soft tissues and to image them in any chosen plane. Sagittal and coronal sections can be made routinely in addition to the conventional axial ones.

9. Conclusions

The limitations of MRI ten years ago related primarily to slice thickness and lack of spatial resolution together with long image acquisition times. Advances in gradient technology and the development of fast spin echo and gradient echo sequences have largely addressed these problems. Continued advances in these areas will lead to the improvement of volume acquisition techniques and the application of echo planar imaging to the lumbar spine. This latter technique allows images to be made in milliseconds and will enable dynamic studies of the spine to be performed.

Every medical student is taught to order investigations to confirm an impression gained from the clinical history and examination. This edict is especially true of MRI which has a well defined place in the investigation of the lumbar spine. Whilst MR imaging remains relatively expensive, it is important that every effort is made to examine those cases in which MRI diagnosis will benefit clinical outcome. It is applicable to those under the age of 20 with unexplained back pain and sciatica and those of any age with sciatic or other neurological signs. It is not considered to be useful in the investigation of uncomplicated back pain, where the demonstration of degenerate and or prolapsed intervertebral discs is of very doubtful significance.

10. References

1. L.A. Aguila, D.W. Piraino, M.T. Modic *et al.*, *Mag. Res. Imag. Radiol.* **155** (1995) 155.
2. D.W.L. Hukins, R.M. Aspden and D.S. Hickey, in *The Biology of the Intervertebral Disc*, Vol. 2 ed. P. Ghosh (CRC Press, Boca Raton, 1988).
3. M.T. Modic and J.S. Ross, *Orthop. Clin. North. Am.* **222** (1991) 283.
4. J.S. Ross, T.J. Masaryk, M.T. Modic *et al.*, *Am. J. Radiol.* **149** (1987) 1025.
5. J.S. Ross, M.T. Modic *et al.*, *Am. J. Neuroradiol.* **10** (1989) 1243.

6.   J.S. Ross, T.J. Masaryk, *et al.*, *Am. J. Neuroradiol* **11** (1990) 771.
7.   S. Yu, B.M. Haughton, L.A. Sether *et al.*, *Radiology* **170** (1989) 523.

CHAPTER 8

DIGITAL VIDEOFLUOROSCOPY AND
ABNORMAL SPINAL MOVEMENT

A.C. Breen and R. Allen

1. Introduction

The scale of the problem of spinal pain is a vast one and much of it relates to understanding the mechanics of the intervertebral holding elements. These structures vary in their responses to load depending on such factors as age, range of movement, bending moment, number of repetitions, duration of force and vertebral level. They must be considered in the context of common life situations such as vibration, prolonged sitting postures and specialised and repeated movements at work. Although basic concepts in mechanics can be utilised to analyse motion and forces in the human body in various activities[12], theoretical considerations fall far short of satisfying the need to understand what happens in life. The pain and disability of spinal dysfunction and injury often does not relate to the degree of apparent damage.

In considering motion and forces in the spine, the greatest progress seems to have been made in researching the latter. Cadaveric specimens often provide satisfactory information with respect to intradiscal pressure[35], connective tissue strength[49] and cellular biophysics[26]. In living subjects, however, the characteristics of holding elements are not accessible for measurement. The relative motions of the vertebrae do, however, reflect these features and research into intervertebral motion *in vivo* is an essential prerequisite for understanding mechanical disorders of the spine.

Our appreciation of motion in the living spine, especially that between individual vertebrae, is largely confined to normal ranges[58] and large increments[10,11]. The use of non-invasive methods such as flexible rulers, inclinometers and goniometers has been well researched[32,34,40,46,56]. Three-dimensional analysis of spinal motion has also been carried out for gross movements using an electromagnetic transmitter/sensor system[41]. These methods recommend themselves where information about the movement of a section of spine, rather than individual segments, is required[20,21,42]. However, the detailed assessment of the kinematics of linkages is a problem requiring measurement from spinal images. In simple terms, the two main considerations are what to measure and how to measure it.

2. Kinematic Indices

The main indices of spinal segmental kinematics were reviewed by White and Panjabi[58] in 1978 and by Frymoyer[15] the following year. These can generally be divided into three groups; those which describe rotations, those which describe translations and those which are made up of both components. The complexity of the subject becomes apparent when all the possible relative motions between selected vertebrae are considered in three dimensions. Not all combinations have practical use, however, and with this in mind, Hoag[25] offered a pragmatic classification of vertebral motion. In addition, and in response to the conflicting terminologies which began to appear, Panjabi, Krag and Goel[38] proposed a three-dimensional co-ordinate system for recording the spatial orientations of vertebrae.

2.1. Motion Studies

Rotational ranges of lateral bending were investigated in normal subjects from X-rays by Tanz[53] and Miles and Sullivan[33]. Further radiographic studies of lateral flexion in the lumbar spine were undertaken by Dimnet *et al.*[10] using digitised anatomical co-ordinates from serial radiographs. These contributed to the establishment of normal *in-vivo* ranges and noted the presence of concurrent paradoxical axial rotations in some subjects (Figure 1). There is no evidence, however, that these are abnormal.

The association between lumbar flexion and back pain has made the study of this plane of motion particularly attractive[52]. The issue of stability and the possibility of damage to discs and posterior joints during flexion led investigators to seek relationships between

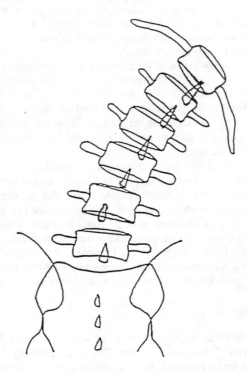

Figure 1. Paradoxical axial rotation at L4 in sidebending.

these problems and this type of motion[1,44,51]. Like lateral flexion, however, the measurement of ranges did not discriminate mechanics related to pain syndromes and the concern of surgeons for the stability of segments focused attention on the measurement of linear displacements, or translations. This was done from X-rays directly. The accuracy of these techniques, which has been reviewed by Schaffer *et al.*[48], is limited mainly by the small size of the movement involved.

Translation has been most successfully described in terms of the position of the instantaneous centre of rotation (ICR) of one bony segment about an adjacent one (Figure 2). The technique, first described by Rosenberg[47], evolved from the application of joint centre analysis to the problem of vertebral motion. Furthermore, the locus, or centrode, of serial increments over the range of intervertebral rotation has been reported normally to be confined to an area of approximately 2 cm diameter within or near the disc space for most spinal levels[19,39].

The length of these centrodes was the first lumbar spine kinematic measure to be associated with pathology[16,17,36,45,50]. Based on samples of live and cadaveric spines, it was proposed that centrode lengths equal to or less than the anterior-posterior dimension of the intervertebral disc (approximately 30 mm in the lumbar spine) are consistent with either normal or very degenerate discs, both of which have inherent stability. Early disc degeneration, however, was associated with larger centrode lengths (over 50 mm) and with suspected vertebral instability.

As can be seen from the above, the literature in respect of lumbar intervertebral motion has been largely confined to considerations of range. Whether rotational or translatory,

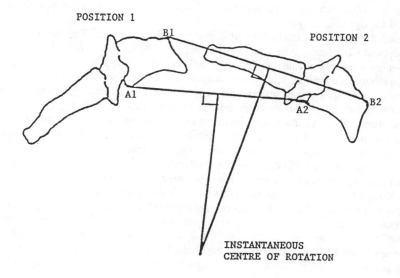

Figure 2. Calculation of the instantaneous centre of rotation (ICR) of a cervical vertebra in the sagittal plane.

normal variation is wide - probably too wide for any meaningful association to be developed with identifiable conditions. To progress beyond this, serial measurement *within* the motion is needed to characterise patterns. Seen in this light, the regularity of intervertebral movement could be quantified, as could the extent to which it is synchronised with other segments. These features can be visualised by viewing X-ray motion sequences using an image intensifier. In order to quantify serial kinematics, however, the videofluoroscopic images must be subjected to digital image processing and measurement.

3. Digital Videofluoroscopy

The use of spinal X-ray images for kinematic assessment was first reported by Todd and Pyle[55] in 1928 and subsequently by Gianturco[18] in 1944 and Hasner[22] in 1952. Since then, the kinematics of the lumbar spine has probably been the most thoroughly investigated of all - sometimes without apparent regard to the hazards of ionising radiation to normal volunteer subjects who underwent extensive serial X-ray studies to establish the ranges of movement. Because of X-ray dosage, few *in-vivo* studies of normal segmental kinematics have been undertaken, most researchers following the example of Hilton, Ball and Benn[24] in using cadaveric lumbar spines. Exceptions are the work of Porter *et al.*[43] and Hibbert *et al.*[23] who used ultrasound to scan the lumbar spine, mainly for canal diameter but also for canal encroachments caused by spondylolisthesis. This method did not give reliable anatomical landmarks for motion analysis but did have the advantage of safety. Magnetic resonance imaging, while non-invasive from the standpoint of radiation, does not, so far, allow full and unencumbered active and passive trunk movement which is essential for dynamic imaging.

Research investigating the validity of digital videofluoroscopy (DVF) was reported in the late 1980's by Breen, Allen and Morris[4-6] and by Cholewicki *et al.*[9]. The technique involves marking co-ordinates on the edges and corners of series of images of vertebrae using an electronic cursor on a computer monitor (Figure 3). The images are obtained by the careful radiography of patients bending, using a modern image intensifier and recorded on videotape for transport to an image processing laboratory.

The programs include algorithms for the calculation of lumbar intervertebral rotations and instantaneous centres of rotation[3]. Work on methods for automatic landmark indentification and tracking is in progress[2]. (These techniques are convertible to MRI should future developments in that technology allow). With modern image intensification, the radiation dosage needed to obtain a lumbar spine motion sequence is less than for a single X-ray of this area and the technique has had some clinical exposure[7].

Line graphs illustrating the progress of intervertebral rotations against time (Figure 4) show that even allowing for error, motion, or the absence of it, is clearly demonstrable. The supposition that the extremes of trunk range also represent the extremes of *intervertebral* range is also dispelled by the method. Lumbar flexion motion from L2 to L5 comparing the changing lumbar angles calculated by an electromagnetic 3-dimensional

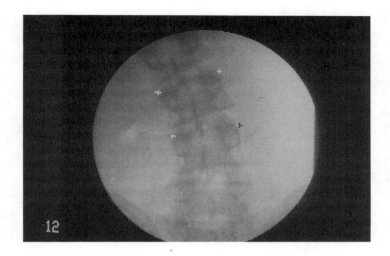

Figure 3. Digitised image from a videofluoroscopic sidebending sequence with electronic landmarks.

inclinometer with DVF showed a poor relationship. This reflects the irregularity of interosseous movements during the comparatively smooth bending of the trunk (Figure 5).

DVF makes possible the demonstration of synchronicity of motion between a series of linkages (Figure 6) but more work will be needed to discover the clinical relevance of

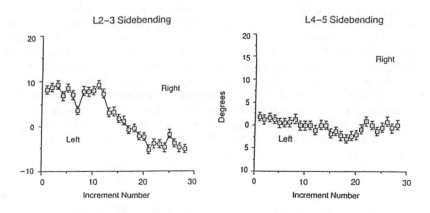

Figure 4. Graphs of sidebending motion sequences showing considerable motion at L2-3 but very little rotation at the L4-5 segment.

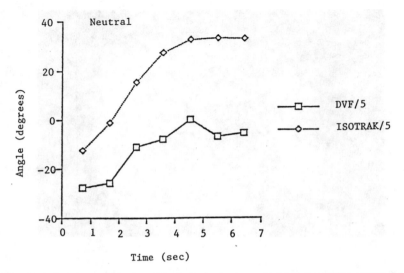

Figure 5. Graph depicting serial lumbar angles in flexion in a normal subject measured by DVF and 3-Space Isotrak.

asynchronous motion. Of more immediate importance is the ongoing concern for lumbar spine instability. Preliminary studies of patients with spinal fusions have demonstrated the technique's ability to discriminate between solid fusions and pseudarthroses to an accuracy of 92 %[31] and could prevent unnecessary second operations.

The concept of stability may also have undergone some refinement. Notwithstanding the importance of overall intervertebral range, what may predispose to disability from moderate day-to-day stresses is the presence of non-elastic, or lax lumbar spine linkages. The load/deformation characteristics of such linkages has been considered in cadaveric spines by Panjabi[37]. If a considerable amount of the intervertebral motion range is covered on minimal loading, this 'neutral zone' of motion is disproportionately large. In kinematic terms, a lax segment will cover most of its range well before the rest of the lumbar spine and this can be quantified using DVF. Preliminary studies have developed an index of laxity which relies on the ratio of the range covered at a linkage within a time interval to that in the lumbar spine as a whole[30]. A Laxity Index above 1.0 therefore suggests relative laxity and below this, relative tension.

4. Conclusion

Quantitative dynamic imaging of the lumbar spine offers the prospect for the assessment of the integrity of these linkages in patients with lumbar spine disorders. Since the Philips Company of Holland developed the first X-ray image intensifier in the 1950's[54],

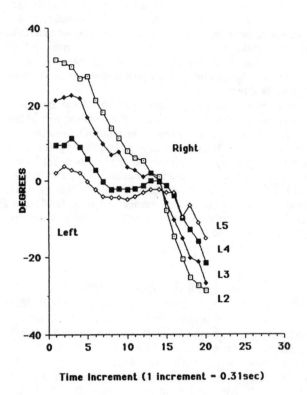

Figure 6. Graph showing synchronicity of L2-5 sidebending motion.

technology has advanced unrecognisably. Even though spine radiologists were slow to adopt the technique, a number[8,13,14,27-29] used it in normal and traumatised living subjects for the subjective assessment of joint motion in the cervical spine.

The prospects for even greater refinements in videofluoroscopic systems are high. Automatic dosage control is already standard, as is image enlargement. A variety of input window sizes are now available and developments in iris, lens control and rectification are being directed towards the reduction of intensifier flare (the tendency to uncontrolled photoelectric emission near the circumference of the input phosphor). Most importantly for patient dosage, unwanted frames within a video sequence can be dispensed with during the examination by pulsing the X-ray beam in synchrony with the camera.

From the viewpoint of joint kinematics, it is the scale of the processing opportunities which appeal. Considering image quality, any improvement in resolution which may be offered by improvements in intensifier design can be taken up by an image processor of sufficient on-line capacity. In terms of enhancement for human appreciation, the manipulation and on-line quantification of grey levels, noise reduction by filtration and edge-finding algorithms all offer the opportunity for more accurate anatomical co-ordinate marking. Geometric distortion brought about either from patient placement, intensifier/camera or computer configuration is amenable to corrective digital transformation[57]. Artificial vision techniques are now being applied to tracking anatomical landmarks through motion sequences.

With the benefits of this technology, abnormal spinal motion can be investigated comprehensively and indices developed. These will extend the role of spine kinematics beyond that of intervertebral ranges and explore the clinical relevance of motion patterns which seem associated with disabilities. Apart from its immediate practical use in assessing patients for whom fusion surgery is contemplated or has failed, DVF can also show the effects of spinal manipulation on intervertebral motion. This could help to explain some of the benefits which the treatment holds for patients with low back pain. The applications of DVF are, however, not unlimited and routine use is to be discouraged. For the foreseeable future, problem patients in well-defined clinical situations will be the beneficiaries of the new technique.

5. References

1.   S.D. Banks, *J. Manip. Physiol. Ther.* **6** (1983) 113.
2.   R. Bilfulco, R. Allen, A. Della Fera, A. De Stefano, R. Magiulo and A.C. Breen, in *Computer Simulations in Biomedicine,* ed. H. Power and R.T. Hart (Computational Mechanics Publications, Southampton, 1995).
3.   A.C. Breen, L. Lapackova, M. Kondracki and R. Allen, *Proc. V. Internat. Symp. Biomed. Eng. (I.F.B.E.)* (1994) 231.
4.   A.C. Breen, R. Allen and A. Morris, *Clin. Biomech.* **3** (1988) 5.
5.   A.C. Breen, R. Allen and A. Morris, *J. Med. Eng. Tech.* **13** (1989) 109.
6.   A.C. Breen, R. Allen and A. Morris, *J. Biomed. Eng.* **11** (1989) 224.
7.   A.C. Breen, R. Brydges, H. Nunn, J. Kause and R. Allen, *Euro. J. Phys. Med. Rehabil.* **3(5)** (1993) 192.
8.   E. Buonocore, J.T. Hartman and C.L. Nelson, *J.A.M.A.* **198** (1966) 25.
9.   J. Cholewicki, S.M. McGill, R.P. Wells and H. Vernon, *Clin. Biomech.* **6** (1991) 73.
10.   J. Dimnet, L.P. Fischer, G. Gonan and J.P. Carret, *J. Biomech.* **11** (1978) 143.
11.   J. Dimnet, A. Pasquet, M.H. Krag and M.M. Panjabi, *J. Biomech.* **15** (1982) 959.
12.   D. Dowson, in *Introduction to the Biomechanics of Joints and Joint Replacement* (Mechanical Engineering Publications Ltd 1981).
13.   J.W. Fielding, *J. Bone Jt Surg.* **39A** (1957) 1280.
14.   J.W. Fielding, *J. Bone Jt Surg.* **46A** (1964) 1779.

15.   J.W. Frymoyer, W.W. Frymoyer, D.G. Wilder and M.H. Pope, *J.Biomech.* **12** (1979) 165.

16.   S.D. Gertzbein, J. Seligman and K. Holtby, *Spine* **4** (1985) 257.

17.   S.D. Gertzbein, R. Holtby, M. Tile, A. Kapasouri, K.W. Chan and B. Cruickshank, *Spine* **9** 409.

18.   C. Gianturco, *Amer. J. Roentgenol.* **52** (1944) 261.

19.   G.P. Gonan, J. Dimnet, J.P. Carret, J.C. de Mauroy, L.P. Fischer and G. De Mourgues, *Acta Orthopaedica Belgica* **48** (1982) 589.

20.   C. Gonnella, S.V. Paris and M. Kutner, *Phys. Ther.* **62** (1982) 62.

21.   F.D. Hart and S.J. Rose, *Proc. I.S.S.L.S.* **7** (1983) 105.

22.   E. Hasner, M. Schalimtzek and E. Snorrason, *Acta Radiol.* **37** (1952) 141.

23.   C.S. Hibbert, C. Delaygue, B. McGlen and R.W. Porter, *Brit. J. Radiol.* **54** (1981) 870.

24.   R.C. Hilton, J. Ball and R.T. Benn, *Ann. Rheum. Dis.* **38** (1979) 378.

25.   J.M. Hoag, M. Kosek and J.R. Moser, *J. Amer. Osteopath. Ass.* **59** (1960) 899.

26.   D.W.L. Hukins, in: *The Lumbar Spine and Back Pain* (3rd edition), ed. M.I.V. Jayson (Longman Group, 1987).

27.   M.D. Jones, *Calif. Med.* **93** (1960) 293.

28.   M.D. Jones, *Amer. J. Roentgenol.* **87** (1962) 1054.

29.   M.D. Jones, *Arch. Surg.* **94** (1967) 206.

30.   M. Kondracki and A.C. Breen, *Proc. Soc. Back Pain. Res.* London (1993).

31.   M. Kondracki, S. Eisenstein, A.C. Breen, R. Williams, *Proc. Soc. Back Pain. Res. Aberdeen* (ARC Publications, 1995).

32.   F.J. Kottke and M.O. Mundale, *Arch. Phys. Med. Rehab.* (1959) 379.

33.   M. Miles, W.E. Sullivan, *Anatomical Record* **139** (1961) 387.

34.   J.M.H. Moll and V. Wright, *Ann. Rheum. Dis.* **30** (1971) 381.

35.   A. Nachemson, in: *The Lumbar Spine and Back Pain* (2nd edition), ed. M.I.V. Jayson (Pitman Medical, 1980).

36.   N.G. Ogston, G.J. King, S.D. Gertzbein, M. Tile, A. Kapasouri and J.D. Rubenstein, *Spine* **11** (1986) 591.

37.   M.M. Panjabi, *J. Spinal Dis.* **5** (1992) 390.

38.   M.M. Panjabi, M.H. Krag, V.K. Goel, *J. Biomech.* **14** (1981) 447.

39.   M.M. Panjabi, M.H. Krag, J.C. Dimnet, S.D. Walter and R.A. Brand, *Orthop.Res.* **1** (1984) 387.

40.   M.J. Pearcy, *Clin. Biomech.* **1** (1986) 44.

41.   M.J. Pearcy and R.J. Hindle, *Clinical Biomech.* **4** (1989) 73.

42.   G.F. Pennel, G.S. Conn, G. McDonald, G. Dale and H. Garside, *J. Bone Jt Surg.* **54B** (1972) 442.

43.   R.W. Porter, M. Wicks and D. Ottewell, *J. Bone Jt Surg.* **60B:2** (1978) 481.

44.   I.R.A. Posner, A.A. White, W.T. Edwards and W.C. Hayes, *Spine* **7** (1982) 374.

45.   S. Reichman, E. Berglund and K. Lundgren, *K.Z. Anat. Entwicklesch* **138** (1972) 283.

46.   T.M.G. Reynolds, *Rheumatol. Rehabil.* **14** (1975) 180.

47.   P. Rosenberg, *J. Amer. Osteo. Ass.* **55** (1955) 103.

48.   W.O. Schaffer, K.F. Spratt, J. Weinstein, T.R. Lehman and V. Goel, *Spine* **15** 741.

49.   A.B. Schultz, D.N. Warwick, M.H. Berkson and A.L. Nachemson, *J. Biomech. Eng.* **101** (1979) 46.

50.   J.V. Seligman, S.D. Gertzbein, M. Tile and A. Kapasouri, *Spine* **9** (1984) 566.

51.   A. Shirazi-Adl, A.M. Ahmed and S.C. Shrivastava, *J. Biomech.* **19** (1986) 331.

52.   I.A.F. Stokes and J.W. Frymoyer, *Spine* **12** (1987) 688.

53.   S.S. Tanz, *Amer. J. Roentgenol.* **69** (1953) 399.

54.   M.C. Teves, *Philips Tech* **17** (1955/6) 69.

55.   T.W. Todd and I.S. Pyle, *Amer. J. Phys. Anthr.* **12** (1928) 321.

56.   J.D.G. Troup, C.A. Hood, and A.E. Chapman, *Ann. Phys. Med.* **9** (1968), 308.

57.   W.A. Wallace and F. Johnson, *J. Biomech.* **14** (1981) 123.

58.   A.A. White and M.M. Panjabi, *Spine* **3** (1978) 12.

CHAPTER 9

RADIONUCLIDE BONE SCANNING

F.W. Smith and P. Thorpe

1. Introduction

In the practice of nuclear medicine, intravenous radioactive nuclides or pharmaceuticals labelled with a radionuclide localise in the organ of interest. This provides information about its size, shape and, more importantly, about its metabolism. Bone scanning is important because diseases which are causing an osteoblastic reaction in bone are visualised long before they are recognised by radiography. It is a highly sensitive method for demonstrating bone disease, often providing an earlier diagnosis and demonstrating more lesions than are found on X-ray. A bone scan demonstrates small changes in bone metabolism, whilst a 50% change in mineral content is necessary for radiological change[1,3.] Bone scan changes occur with increased blood flow or increased osteoblastic activity. Even though the appearances of lesions are non-specific, bone scanning often helps in back pain diagnosis, especially when combined with the clinical history and other investigations.

Bone scanning is currently used to investigate a wide range of spinal disorders, both benign and malignant, in adults and children. It is important that the clinician is able to recognise the normal appearances, and variations in both the adult and immature skeleton.

2. Radiopharmaceuticals

Technetium-99m-labelled phosphates and phosphonate analogues are widely used today. Strontium-85, Strontium-87, Fluorine-18 and Gallium-67 are unsatisfactory because of either high radiation doses or poor imaging characteristics. Most 99mTc phosphate compounds have low radiation doses. They emit gamma rays and no beta particles and they have a short radioactive half-life of 6 h. A number of phosphate analogues are available, of which methylene diphosphonate (MDP) is probably the most useful[6]. These diphosphonates are stable *in vivo*, having, like pyrophosphate, their phosphorus bound to carbon rather than to oxygen. They are, therefore, more rapidly cleared from the soft tissues. They give a high bone to soft tissue ratio 2-3 h after administration. Of the injected dose, 50-60% localises in bone, and the remainder is excreted by the kidneys.

A number of factors influence the uptake of 99mTc-labelled diphosphonate by bone, especially the blood supply and rate of bone turnover. Others include the quantity of mineralised bone, capillary permeability, local acid-base balance, the fluid pressure within bone, vitamins and hormones. Diphosphonate probably first binds to the bone by adsorption and then to the crystalline lattice of the calcium hydroxyapatite and organic matrix, but the precise mechanism of uptake is unknown.

3. Imaging method

Conventional or delayed images are usually obtained with a gamma camera 3-4 h following the intravenous injection of 500 MBq (15 mCi) 99mTc-labelled MDP. However, when infection or inflammation of a bone or joint is suspected, or when the assessment of blood flow to a region is required, it is necessary to perform a three-phase examination. The region of interest in the spine is first placed under the camera prior to the intravenous injection and then, following a bolus injection, a series of 2-s images is taken for a duration of 1 min. The second phase is obtained 5 minutes later demonstrating a blood pool image of the areas of hyperaemia in the bone, joints or soft tissue. Thirdly, the AP and oblique views of the spine and the rest of the skeleton are taken 3-4 h later, after emptying the urinary bladder. The urinary tract is the main route of excretion of 99mTc MDP. Although bone scans are extremely sensitive at localising abnormalities in the skeleton, they are non-specific for the cause of the increased uptake of radionuclide. Diagnostic accuracy is improved by comparing the bone scan with relevant radiographs.

4. The normal bone scan

A good knowledge of the normal appearances and normal variations of bone scans avoids interpretative error. The bone scan shows less anatomical detail than conventional radiographs but the vertebral bodies and the transverse processes of the lumbar and lower dorsal spine are easily recognised. It is less easy to identify them in the upper dorsal and cervical spine (Figure 1). The ribs and scapulae are clearly seen, and the pelvis is recognised with a relatively higher uptake in both sacroiliac joints and less in the sacrum and coccyx. The thoracic and lumbar lordosis affects the appearance of the scan because of the proximity of the vertebrae to the detector. The lumbar vertebrae may appear more intense and in focus whilst the dorsal vertebrae being further from the detector are less intense and blurred. The rotation of a scoliosis may erroneously suggest a high uptake in some pedicles. There is a high uptake of radiopharmaceutical in the epiphyses of children and adolescents because of the naturally high metabolic activity in the developing epiphyses. Approximately 50% of the injected dose of radiopharmaceutical is excreted by the kidneys, and the urinary tract is therefore well visualised. An unsuspected urinary tract obstruction may be diagnosed from the bone scan as a cause of back pain, and sometimes a renal tumour may be seen with metastases from a hypernephroma[7]. Uptake may also be increased in the soft tissue metastases of liver or lung, after a recent infarct of heart or brain, in some leaking wounds[4] and in the normal female breast.

5. The abnormal bone scan

5.1. Neoplastic disease
Radiopharmactuticals accumulate in primary bone tumours, but this is a non-specific finding because similar appearances exist in both malignant and benign bone tumours, in

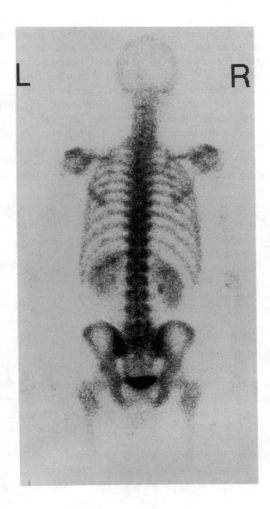

Figure 1. Normal posterior view bone scan.

infection and healing fractures. It has no value beyond demonstrating the site and extent of the tumour. Bone scans can be used to estimate the extent of a primary bone tumour, but this has largely been superseded by magnetic resonance imaging (MRI) which shows the full extent of the lesion. Bone scanning has value, therefore, only in discovering the presence of the tumour as a cause of back pain.

Benign primary bone tumours of the appendicular skeleton, such as osteoid osteoma, are usually easy to identify on conventional radiographs, but they may be difficult to detect in the spine[8]. Bone scans can localise these tumours in the spine in the absence of radiological change[2]. The appearances of osteoid osteoma are usually characteristic (Figure 2), but they can at times be confused with other benign conditions such as aneurysmal bone cyst and haemangioma which may be very similar to an osteoid osteoma. In the delayed 4-h image the tumour appears as a small area of very intense uptake, usually in an appendage of a vertebra. The earlier blood pool image also shows a discrete area of high uptake which matches that of the later image. It is important, therefore, always to take both a blood pool and delayed image in all patients with unexplained back ache. It is then possible to differentiate osteoid osteoma from some other cause of back pain such as spondylolisthesis which may show the same appearances in the late images but not on the

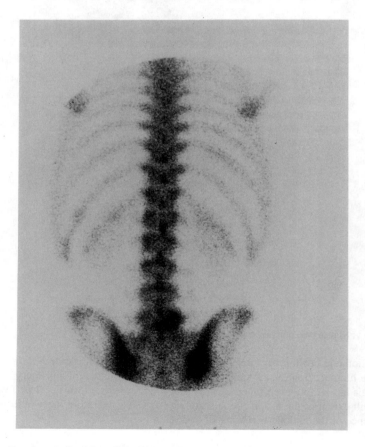

Figure 2. Osteoid osteoma in the right pedicle of L5 vertebra

blood pool image[5].

Perhaps the most common indication for bone scanning is the investigation of bone metastases in patients with a known or suspected primary carcinoma. It is often possible to demonstrate the presence and extent of such lesions. It has been well recognised for over 20 years that radionuclide bone scans can demonstrate bone metastases long before they are visible on X-ray. Osteoblastic metastases show as areas of high uptake in bone (Figure 3) and, whilst their appearances are usually non-specific for the nature of the primary tumour, it is often possible to be specific about secondaries from prostatic carcinoma. The uptake in bone metastases from prostatic carcinoma is very dense, often with a uniform uptake in each vertebral body. The appearance may vary from three or four discrete deposits of high uptake to uniform involvement of the entire skeleton, the so called superscan. It may be difficult to differentiate prostatic metastases from Paget's disease when only the vertebral bodies are involved, since both conditions show exceptionally high uptake of 99mTc-MDP. When other bones such as the pelvic bones, skull or long bones are also affected by Paget's disease the differentiation from metastases is easier (Figure 4),

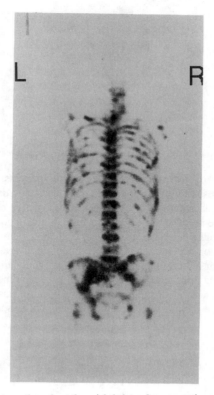

Figure 3. Widespread metastases throughout the axial skeleton from prostatic carcinoma.

though the two conditions may co-exist. The bone scan will demonstrate osteoblastic metastases earlier than X-rays, and also give a more accurate description of their number, size and activity.

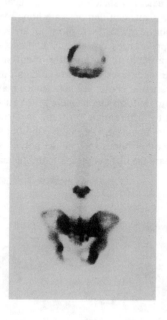

Figure 4. Characteristic appearances of Paget's disease involving L3, the pelvis and skull.

One or two areas of increased uptake, even in patients with known primary malignancy, may be caused by pathology other than metastatic disease. X-rays of these areas should be examined carefully to exclude fracture, active degenerative change or Paget's disease. The false-negative rate of bone scans in detecting bone metastases is small, mainly in patients with highly anaplastic carcinoma, or in those with slow-growing tumours with relatively little osteoblastic reaction. Osteolytic metastases are not usually discernible until they are more than 2-3 cm in diameter, when they show areas of absent uptake of 99mTc-MDP (Figure 5). Bone scanning is therefore not recommended in the search for osteolytic carcinoma metastases or multiple myeloma because small deposits may not be demonstrated. Even with widespread multiple myeloma the bone scan may appear entirely normal.

5.2. Trauma

Fractures of the vertebral bodies give positive images on bone scans which usually appear as linear areas of increased uptake (Figure 6). The concentration of the

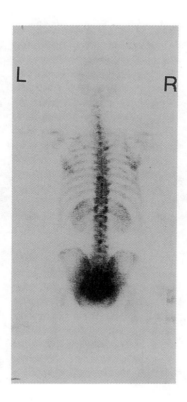

Figure 5. Mixed osteoblastic and osteolytic metastases.

radiopharmaceutical increases for 6 months at the sites of recent fractures, but then slowly decreases as healing progresses. Thus, recent fractures less than 6 months old show a more intense uptake than older ones. The bone scan is a valuable method for determining the age of vertebral compression fractures in osteoporotic patients, but it cannot distinguish between benign and malignant causes of vertebral body compression.

A bone scan can clearly demonstrate stress fractures as areas of increased bone activity. Recent and healing fractures are well demonstrated at 4 h but do not show on the blood pool image, whereas osteoid osteomas, haemangiomas and infection show on both. A negative scan does not exclude an established spondylolisthesis, but it excludes stress fracture of the pars inter-articularis. A positive scan suggests potential for healing. It is particularly valuable in the early lesion of spondylolysis. The patient should be treated as having a stress fracture in order to prevent an established spondylolisthesis and possible long-term disability.

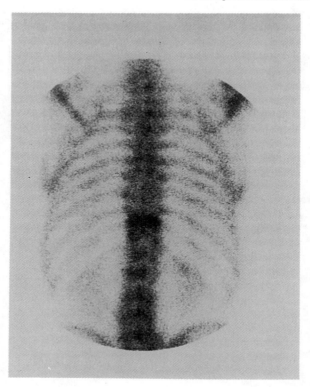

Figure 6. Recent Compression fracture of D11 vertebra.

5.3. Infection

Osteomyelitis of the spine can be demonstrated by bone scanning. It shows both increased uptake in the blood pool images as a result of increased blood flow to the infected bone, and also intense uptake in the later images. When both blood pool and late views are made the diagnosis is usually not in doubt. If, however, only late images are made then it is necessary to correlate the clinical history and X-rays with the bone scan to differentiate infection from other pathology. Osteomyelitis can be distinguished from cellulitis by using both blood pool and late images. Osteomyelitis generally shows increased vascularity and increased bone activity appearing in both phases of examination, whilst cellulitis shows increased vascularity adjacent to bone in the blood pool phase, and little or no increase in bone uptake in the late images.

Occasionally acute osteomyelitis does not show as an area of high uptake but as a 'cold' area. This paradoxical appearance is not understood, but may be due to thrombosis of medullary vessels and relative ischaemia. This finding is seen only in the first few days of the disease. It is more common in young children and is unusual in the spine, probably because the diagnosis of vertebral osteomyelitis is sometimes delayed.

5.4. Arthritic and degenerative conditions

Because bone scanning can demonstrate increased vascularity and increased bone activity, it has a place in the investigation of degenerative joint disease. It can define the extent of active disease and distinguish between acute active and chronic degenerative changes. Chronic osteoarthritis appears as an ill-defined loss of definition of the joint space. Active disease shows an ill-defined boundary but also a diffuse increase in activity (Figure 7). This is less intense than is seen in healing fractures, malignancy or infection. Bone scanning can document the early presence of arthritis and assess serial changes in the disease, but it has not been tested in facet joint arthritis.

In the active phase of ankylosing spondylitis certain characteristic features may be seen on a bone scan. There is often an increase in uptake in the costo- vertebral joints of the dorsal spine giving the so called 'pine tree' appearance. This is not usually seen during remission. There may also be a significant increase in uptake in the sacroiliac joints. Attempts to assess the severity of disease by quantifying this increased uptake have not shown practical value.

Sacroiliitis is better diagnosed by bone scan than X-ray, since radiographs are seldom positive at an early stage in this disease. Both blood pool and later images are positive, but it may be difficult to differentiate an infective from an inflammatory condition. In osteitis condensans ilii the bone scan will not be positive, which will help to differentiate it from

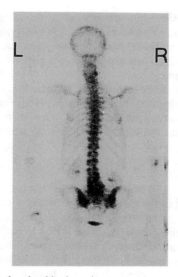

Figure 7. Osteoarthritis of cervical, dorsal and lumbar spine.

sacroiliitis. Patients with Scheuermann's disease do not show bone scan abnormalities at any stage of the disease. An abnormal bone scan would suggest some other disease process.

5.5. Metabolic bone disease

The precise role for bone scanning in metabolic bone disease has not been defined. However, there are certain characteristic features which, if seen during the scanning of patients with unexplained back pain, might suggest a metabolic bone disorder. Primary and secondary hyper-parathyroidism may both produce increased osteoblastic activity. It may be demonstrated as a generally high uptake throughout the entire skeleton, with increased bone to soft tissue contrast. Alternatively there may be increased uptake in the endplates of the vertebrae mimicking the radiographic 'rugger jersey' appearance. These changes should lead to an examination of the chest and skull. The latter is likely to show increased calvarial uptake and the sternum to show a higher uptake than the ribs, the so-called 'tie' sign. There will also be an absence of the normal renal activity. Brown tumours do not accumulate 99mTc-MDP.

No significant abnormality in bone uptake is seen in patients with primary osteoporosis because the bone scan is not sensitive enough to show any general decrease in uptake. However, focal abnormalities may be seen in these patients as a result of everyday minor trauma and microfractures.

In osteomalacia there is a rapid uptake of tracer after injection and a high bone to soft tissue ratio. Fractures and pseudofractures show as small areas of intense activity and must be differentiated from metastatic disease. This is not difficult because in osteomalacia the rib lesions tend to involve a number of adjacent ribs in line.

5.6. Other bone disorders

The bone scan is sensitive but non-specific in detecting osteoblast activity. Positive bone scans will be found in fibrous dysplasia, non-ossifying fibroma, osteochondroma, benign osteoblastoma, lymphoma, haemangioma, sarcoma, eosinophilic granuloma, the healing phase of avascular necrosis and fractures in patients with osteogenesis imperfecta or the child abuse syndrome.

No increase in uptake will be seen in bone islands. Focal areas of decreased or absent uptake can be seen if they are relatively large. They may be present in metastatic malignancy, early post-traumatic aseptic necrosis, bone infarct, sickle cell crisis, myeloma and eosinophilic granuloma, leukaemia and following radiotherapy.

6. Conclusions

Bone scanning with 99mTc-labelled phosphates thus provides a sensitive, non-invasive method for the detection of a wide variety of diseases affecting the spine. These include traumatic, inflammatory, neoplastic, metabolic and degenerative causes. The bone scan will show osteoblastic changes long before X-rays will show any increase in calcium content, and will detect many diseases weeks or months before any changes are evident radiologically. The relatively poor resolution of the bone scan adds to its poor specificity and X-rays are essential for accurate diagnosis. Bone scan complements X-rays and is a diagnostic procedure which should be considered in patients with back pain because when read in conjunction with the relevant X-rays it will improve patient management.

7. References

1. J. Borak, *Surg. Gynaec. Obstet.* **75** (1942) 599.
2. D.L. Gilday and J.M. Ash. *Sem. Nucl. Med.* **6** (1976) 33.
3. G. Simon, In *Principles of bone X-ray diagnosis.* (Butterworths, London 1973).
4. F.W. Smith. In *Practical Nuclear Medicine*, eds. P.F. Sharp, H.G. Gemmell and F.W. Smith (IRL Press, Oxford, 1989) p. 245.
5. F.W. Smith and D.L. Gilday, *Radiology* **137** (1980) 191.
6. G. Subramanian, J.G. McAfee, R.J. Blair, F.A. Kallfetz and F.D. Thomas. *J. Nucl. Med.* **16** (1975) 744.
7. F. Vieras and C.M. Boyd, *J. Nucl. Med.* **16** (1975) 1109.
8. P.F. Winter, P.M. Johnson, S.K. Hilal and F. Feldman. *Radiology* **122** (1977) 177.

CHAPTER 10

SPONDYLOLISTHESIS

J.R. Johnson

1. Introduction

Although Kilian is credited with the first description of spondylolisthesis in 1854, slipping of the 4th or 5th lumbar vertebra had been described by Herbineaux - a Belgian Obstetrician in the 18th Century and by Rokitansky in 1839. However, it was Neugebauer[20] in 1888 who first recognised the congenital defect of the pars interarticularis as a cause. Meyerding[19], in 1932, confirmed this finding and suggested posterior fusion as the ideal form of treatment for severe symptoms of spondylolisthesis.

In 1963, Newman[21] stressed the dangers of attempted reduction by traction before fusion and made the first attempt to classify the disorder. Under the auspices of the International Society for the Study of the Lumbar Spine this classification was modified by Newman in conjunction with Wiltse and McNab in 1973 and this is now the internationally recognised classification[28].

2. Classification

1. Dysplastic. In these cases there is congenital deficiency of the superior sacral or inferior 5th lumbar facets or both these. This condition is more common in females (approximately 3:2).

2. Isthmic. The typical spondylolytic defect in the pars interarticularis permitting forward slipping of the 5th lumbar vertebra. More common in males. Is subdivided into 3 types:
(a) Lytic - a fatigue fracture of the pars.
(b) Elongated (attenuated) but intact pars.
(c) Acute fracture.

3. Degenerative. Due to failure of the disc and facet joints with degeneration and usually occurs at L4/5.

4. Traumatic. Caused by acute fractures in the area of the pedicle or lamina.

5. Pathological. Attenuation of the pedicle due to tumour or weakness of the bone, *eg.* osteo-genesis.

Classically the clinical syndrome of spondylolisthesis relates to types 1 and 2 which occur in children in adolescence. The difference between type 1 and type 2 may be indistinct. However, children with type 1 spondylolisthesis tend to slip more frequently and have more persistent symptoms than type 2.

The role of genetic factors in the development of lumbar spondylolisthesis has been agreed by many authors despite the fact that lumbar spondylolisthesis has not been seen in new born infants on X-ray examination. The slip normally develops during the growth period and the incidence in the adult population is around 5-6%. In a recent study of patients with a symptomatic slip of 50% or more, there was a 4-fold prevalence in relatives of the subjects compared with the normal population. It has also been suggested that there is an increased prevalence in gymnasts and ballet dancers indicating that trauma may also be a prominent factor in the aetiology.

Major degrees of slipping occur in the dysplastic type. Children in this group slip more frequently and have more persistent symptoms than patients in type 2b. Hensinger[13] found that 40% of his patients that required surgery came from type 1 - the dysplastic group. The lytic types rarely have a displacement of more than 30%. This is the group that appears to be 4 times more common in gymnasts and also in weight lifters.

3. Measurement of slip

Recognition of the type of slip and degree of slip is important because of the prognostic significance. Over the years various attempts have been made to measure the degree of deformity. It should be remembered that in children and adolescents the degree of slip may change with flexion and extension and there may be a difference between supine and standing views. In adults the degree of slip is not usually altered by body position.

Two types of measurement have been described.

1. Tangential or forward displacement - (usually known as the Meyerding method). The AP diameter of the superior surface of the 1st sacral vertebra is divided into quarters and the slip of L5 is assigned a grade of 1,2,3 or 4 respectively.

A more precise method is that of Taillard (modified by Boxall[2]) which uses a percentage slip. The tangential or forward displacement is determined by measuring the distance from the back of the 1st sacral vertebra to the back or the posterior border of the 5th lumbar vertebra and dividing this by the AP dimension of the inferior surface of the 5th lumbar vertebra. This is expressed as a percentage slip.

2. Angular slip or sagittal rotation - the angular slip is measured by drawing a line parallel to the inferior surface of the 5th lumbar vertebra and another drawn perpendicular to the posterior aspect of the 1st sacral vertebra. It is the slip angle that probably is the most relevant in terms of cosmetic deformity and is the one measurement that seems to have some prognostic use with regard to the liability of a further slip.

4. Dysplastic spondylolisthesis

Dysplastic spondylolisthesis is unstable until several years after puberty. Symptoms are relatively uncommon in children and are not usually severe enough in teenage years to require medical attention. Symptoms are often decreased by rest and limitation of activities. Females are more prone to severe displacement and therefore present earlier with an increasing deformity and increasing symptoms. Although they have a lower overall incidence, they are more likely to require surgical treatment. Many children may present with no pain but with a postural or gait abnormality. Instability seems to cause hamstring and spinal muscle spasm and this limits forward flexion and gives tight hamstrings with a decreased straight leg raise. Neurological symptoms are uncommon even with an extreme displacement but tight hamstrings may be found with any grade of slip.

The classic clinical presentation is that of the 'lumbar crisis', probably due to a sudden extreme displacement. This gives marked lumbar pain occasionally with some sciatic radiation and extreme limitation of spinal flexion and straight leg raising. The resultant picture is of a bizarre posture with a flexed spine and knees due to the tight hamstrings. The patients walk with an awkward waddling gait.

5. Isthmic spondylolisthesis

The cause of this type of slip is a defect in the pars, probably due to repeated minor trauma and it is a far more common type of disorder than the dysplastic variety. This group have normal facet joints, the problems are due to a spondylolysis, and therefore the slip is rarely more than 30%. It commonly occurs at L5 or occasionally at L4 but can occur at any lumbar level or even at multiple levels. If it presents clinically (and it may not) the commonest presentation is in young people in the late teens and early 20's. This may be because the pars are thin and are not fully mature until approximately this age. There is often a family history and there is an increased incidence in patients with Scheuermann's disease.

As already mentioned there is a higher incidence of the defect in gymnasts, which would suggest that there is a developmental defect during adolescence which may be related to a stress fracture[14,17].

5.1. Clinical presentation
These patients usually present after puberty complaining of lumbo-sacral backache which is made worse by standing or by sporting activities. On examination there is often excellent forward flexion but some discomfort on extending from the flexed position. There is often some discomfort on straight leg raising with occasionally a palpable step or tenderness.

5.2. Spondylolysis without slip
Frederickson in 1984 in a long term follow-up of 500 unselected children over a 25 year period found that the incidence of spondylolysis with or without a slip was 4.4% at the age of 6 compared with an incidence of 6% in adults[10]. He found that the progression of slip was unlikely to increase beyond adolescence and confirmed an earlier report by Blackburn and Velikas that a slip of 30% of less at presentation was unlikely to progress to over 30%[1]. Very few of Frederickson's patients came to surgery or even developed

backache as adults. Spondylolysis without slip is rarely symptomatic in adolescence and therefore other causes of pain should be looked for in cases presenting with back pain.

Spondylolysis of L4 and above is more common in young adults rather than adolescence and at L4 is often associated with partial or complete sacralisation of L5. This condition is much more common in males and the cause would appear to be more traumatic than due to hypoplasia. This group of patients are more likely to get neurological problems of lateral canal stenosis and may require decompression and/or fusion.

6. Investigations

6.1. Plain X-rays

These should show the spondylolysis as a radio-lucent defect in the pars. However, about 20% of defects may be missed if only AP and lateral films are taken and therefore oblique views are essential in the diagnosis of this condition. The AP view will reveal other segmental anomalies which are common such as spina bifida occulta and combinations of sacralisation and lumbarisation. The lateral view is used for looking at the basic lesion of the slip, the normality or otherwise of the lumbo-sacral facet joint and whether there is elongation or lysis of the pars. Often the L5 vertebra is trapezoidal in shape and if this is associated with a dome shaped surface of S1 the patient is more prone to further slippage and deformity.

6.2. Bone scanning

May be useful in the diagnosis of hair line spondylolytic fractures in sporting injuries. It is also useful to establish healing in patients treated conservatively and for diagnosing other lesions such as an osteoid osteoma, infection or malignancy in the differential diagnosis (see Chapter 9).

6.3. CT scanning

This may not always be helpful as the axial cuts through the L5/S1 area may miss the defect. In adult cases with an established defect, CT scanning may be help to outline the mass of the pseudoarthrosis if the patient is complaining of neurological symptoms[18].

6.4. MRI scanning

MRI is helpful during planning for surgery, looking particularly for disc degeneration in the disc above the spondylolisthesis which needs to be taken into account when planning surgical procedures such as fusion. (See also Chapter 7).

6.5. Myelography

This should not be necessary in children but in adults may be helpful in patients where there are symptoms of root compression by delineating the exact level and area of any root entrapment.

7. Treatment of spondylolisthesis

An adult found to have a lytic defect but with no symptoms can probably be reassured that they should be able to lead a normal life and no particular restrictions should be applied. If the patient is not skeletally mature, then it is reasonable to keep the patient under review with occasional X-rays until they have stopped growing and they perhaps should be advised to avoid sports such as gymnastics, cricket *etc*.

If there is a degree of slip but no particular symptoms, then it would seem sensible to advise patients to be careful and sensible with their sporting activities and work. There have been papers to suggest that the L5/S1 disc is likely to become degenerate at an earlier age in patients with a lytic defect and it may also predispose to earlier failure of the disc above. However, once the patient is skeletally mature there is no risk of any further slip and therefore patients in this group should be treated symptomatically.

If the patient presents with backache then conservative measures with back strengthening exercises for the abdominal and back muscles may be all that is necessary. In cases of more severe symptoms then a period of bed rest followed by a plaster cast or orthosis may be useful. In the young athlete where there is the suggestion that there is a pars fracture, then there should be a period of rest to allow the fracture to heal followed by a plaster jacket and possibly a bone scan to see if there is a stress fracture which will heal with conservative treatment.

Young adults who present with back pain and either no slip or a minimal slip which do not settle with conservative treatment, may be advised to have surgical repair of the spondylolisthetic defect. This can be done either by the Buck technique with screws across the defect[4], or the Edinburgh technique with clearance of the defect and a local graft . These techniques are particularly useful in the levels above L5. At L5 the Buck technique can sometimes be used or, alternatively, a straight-forward lateral mass fusion has a good success rate[27]. The techniques of surgical repair should not be used in patients who already have a degenerate disc.

8. Treatment of spondylolisthesis in the adolescent

8.1. Asymptomatic

Many children with spondylolisthesis never get symptoms[28]. If patients are picked up on routine screening, the treatment should depend on the percentage slip on presentation. If the slip is less than 25% there would appear to be no necessity for any particular restrictions for the reasons given above. Over 25% then the patient should be advised to restrict their sporting activities and should be monitored until they are skeletally mature.

8.2. Symptomatic

The main indications for treatment are pain and disability rather than the actual deformity. There are certain risk factors for continued pain, deformity or progression. These factors include an early onset in terms of age, the female sex, recurrent episodes of back pain and a postural deformity or abnormal gait on presentation. As already mentioned under the heading of radiological investigation, there are also certain radiological risk factors. Patients are more likely to progress if they have a type 1 rather than a type 2 slip, if the degree of slip is more than 50% on first presentation and, perhaps more importantly, if they have a high slip angle.

Treatment, therefore, depends to a certain degree on the level of the slip on presentation and on symptoms. With the lower degrees of slip, patients presenting with some pain can be treated conservatively by rest and bracing. However, unless this resolves the symptoms then surgery may be indicated. Radiographs are normally taken every 6 months, particularly covering the adolescent growth spurt period. Generally, if symptoms persist or if there is an increasing slip, then a one level lateral mass fusion is performed.

8.3. Lumbar Crisis at or around puberty

If a patient presents with a clinical lumbar crisis, a lateral mass fusion will normally suffice if the displacement is less than 50%. Over 50% there may be some indication to reduce or fix (see below).

9. Operative treatment of spondylolisthesis

9.1. Fusion in situ

Up until the 1970's most authors agreed that a posterior or postero-lateral inter-transverse fusion was the treatment of choice for children, even those with severe symptoms from spondylolisthesis[5,28]. However, in the 80's there was a series of papers which suggested that attempts should be made to reduce the spondylolisthesis in order to improve the height of the patient and the appearance of the back, and also because of the supposed incidence of non-unions and continuing post-operative slip.

In slips under 50% the cosmetic deformity is minimal and therefore reduction is not indicated. Non-union and a slight slip post-operatively is compatible with a very satisfactory clinical result and there have now been several papers suggesting that fusion *in situ* is very satisfactory for these patients[15,24,26]. Others have suggested anterior fusion without reduction as an alternative, although the complication rate of this is likely to be higher[11].

9.2. The anterior approach

May be used as a primary procedure but might also be useful as a salvage procedure in patients whose postero-lateral fusion has been complicated by non-union or post-operative slip[3,16].

9.3. Reduction and fusion

With major slips greater than 50% or with the spondylolisthetic crisis, it has been suggested that re-positioning the vertebra might be expected to improve the fusion rate. This involves a combined anterior and posterior approach with anterior fusion and stabilisation usually with an implant posteriorly. Initially, Boxall[2] reported internal fixation with Harrington instrumentation. However, reduction was often not maintained and 3 of his patients had major complications. Several other authors reported either minor and transient neurological complications or some serious and permanent ones[2,6,8,12,25].

A review of Newman's patients in 1983 show that even after a severe spondylolisthesis, a good result was obtained with fusion *in situ* and that the spasm abnormal gait and even scoliosis seem to disappear when the fusion becomes solid. In this group an acceptable cosmetic result was achieved in over 90% of the patients followed-up for up to 20 years after their operation[15].

Another long term follow-up in 1989 by Freeman and Donate also confirm that intra-transverse fusion without reduction yielded an acceptable cosmetic result.

9.4. Closed reduction followed by fusion

Because of the neurological problems of open reduction, attempts have been made to reduce the slip angle using extension and traction pre-operatively and, after achieving suitable reduction, the patients are then fused using the postero-lateral technique, usually with fixation. However, even using this technique there have been some causes of at least transient radiculopathy.

More recent techniques involve a slow, controlled reduction, intra-operatively, and it may be that one of these methods may prove to be safe. However, in patients with dysplastic spondylolisthesis, the L5 roots may be shortened by the chronic displacement and it may not be possible to reduce these vertebrae which are already abnormally shaped without any risk to the nerves. At this time, therefore, attempted reduction of severe spondylolisthesis remains a controversial topic.

10. Spondylolisthesis in the older age group

Patients over the age of 35 presenting with back pain and or sciatica require further investigations to try to find the cause of their symptoms. As spondylolytic defects occur in about 5% of the population, other causes of back pain and sciatica should be excluded before ascribing the cause to the pars defect. Ideally an MRI scan is the investigation of choice to look at the disc status and evidence for nerve root compression at the level of the slip or above it. Failing this, radiculography or CT scanning at least should be carried out before making any decisions.

At L5, nerve root compression from the pseudoarthrosis mass can be treated by simple decompression. If the symptom is back pain and there is merely a degenerate disc, then an inter-transverse fusion will suffice.

At levels above L5 the spondylolisthesis may progress as the disc degenerates. It is therefore necessary to assess disc height before making any decisions. If the symptoms are merely those of sciatica, a decompression may suffice when the disc is already degenerate and it is felt that the slip will not progress. However, in a patient with a normal disc height one can expect the spondylolisthesis to progress slightly as the disc degenerates and in these patients a fusion, probably with instrumentation, is indicated in addition to the decompression. In cases of back pain, defects above L5 do not behave the same way as at L5 and are more likely to need fusion than conservative treatment[14].

11. Degenerative spondylolisthesis

Degenerative spondylolisthesis is a distinct clinical entity characterised by degenerative changes in the facet joints and the disc. Erosion and remodelling of the facet joints allows slipping of the vertebra. Because there is not a true spondylolisthetic defect the slip is never more than about 25% and, as in lateral canal stenosis, it is the root emerging below the level of the spondylolisthesis which causes symptoms, *i.e.* an L4/5 degenerative spondylolisthesis, which is the commonest level, presents with L5 root symptoms and signs.

The typical history of these patients is one of a long history of back pain, often a decade or more with a gradual and insidious onset of radicular leg pain and/or neurogenic claudication. It is more common in women and occurs most frequently at L4/5 followed by L3/4 and L5/S1.

The pain is typically worse on walking and standing and is relieved by sitting. Examination is often unhelpful and these patients have full straight leg raising and rarely any objective neurological signs. Occasionally patients present with a heaviness or weakness of the legs, again particularly on walking.

The differential diagnosis is from vascular claudication and often the two conditions may coexist making the diagnosis difficult.

11.1. Treatment of degenerative spondylolisthesis

Initially, conservative treatment, particularly if the patient has back pain, may be sufficient. Lumbar corsets can be helpful. Physiotherapy also may help and some patients will respond to the injection of Calcitonin[23]. Many patients also respond to epidural injections of local anaesthetic and cortisone.

In view of the differential diagnosis from vascular claudication and occasionally from osteo-arthritis in the hips, investigation is mandatory before surgery. The investigation of choice as an initial screening tool is the MRI scan but if this shows multiple levels of narrowing, it may be necessary to perform the 'gold standard' of radiculography combined with CT scanning. The symptoms usually originate from the most severe level of stenosis and surgery at one level is often sufficient to relieve the patient's symptoms. It is not necessary to do multiple level wide laminectomies. Surgery should be confined to decompression of the appropriate compressed root and this can be performed using a localised decompressive technique at each level leaving the mid-line structures intact. Having achieved an adequate root decompression, a decision has to be made as to whether to combine this with a fusion. If the disc is already degenerate then no further slip is likely to occur and it may be sufficient to decompress alone. However, if there is a good disc height, it is likely that the vertebra will slip anteriorly as the disc degenerates further and these patients may get further symptoms if they are not fused. Fusion is obviously a more major procedure for the elderly patient and good results from a decompression alone are often achieved[7,9].

If a decision has been made to fuse at a level above L5, then it may be advisable to combine fusion with pedicular fixation. The results of recent meta-analyses seem to support this clinical impression and it would seem that spinal fusion with instrumentation does enhance fusion rates and improve patient satisfaction in terms of results.

Anterior fusion can also be used and good results have been claimed for anterior fusion without decompression or even combined anterior and posterior fusion without decompression. The rationale for this is correction of deformity and re-establishing the disc height, presumably with some stretching of the ligamentum flavum which is often producing the compression. Again this would seem a rather aggressive approach to patients who are often elderly and medically unfit.

12. References

1. J.S. Blackburn and E.P. Velikas, *J. Bone Joint Surg.* **59-B** (1977) 490.
2. D. Boxall, D.S. Bradford, R.B. Winter and J.H. Moe, *J. Bone Joint Surg.* **61-A** (1979) 479.
3. D.S. Bradford and Y. Gotfried, *J. Bone Joint Surg.* **69-A** (1987) 191.
4. J.E. Buck, *J.Bone Joint Surg.* **52-B** (1970) 432.
5. D.J. Dandy and M.J. Shannon, *J. Bone Joint Surg.* **53-B** (1971) 578.
6. R.I. Dewald, M.M. Faut, R.F. Tadonio and M.C. Neuwirth, *J. Bone Joint Surg.* **63-A** (1981) 619.
7. A. Deburge, B. Lassale, M. Benoist and J. Cauchoix, *Rev. Rheum. Mal. Osteoarc.* **50** (1983) 47.
8. W.T. Dick and B. Schnebel, *Clin. Orthop.* **232** (1988) 79.
9. N.E. Epstein, J.A. Epstein, R. Carras and Lavine L S *Neurosurgery* **13** (1983) 555.
10. B.E. Frederickson, D. Baker, W.J. McHolic, H.A. Yua and J.P. Lubicky, *J. Bone Joint Surg.* **66-A** (1984) 699.
11. D. Freebody, R. Bendall and R.D. Taylor, *J.Bone Joint Surg.* **53-B** (1971) 617.
12. G.R. Harrington and J.H. Dickson, *Clin. Orthop.* **117** (1976) 157.
13. R.N. Hensinger, *J. Bone Joint Surg.* **71-A** (1989) 1098.
14. A.M. Jackson, E. Kirwan and M. Sullivan *J. Bone Joint Surg.* **60-B** (1978) 439.
15. J.R. Johnson and E.O. Kirwan *J. Bone Joint Surg.* **65-B** (1983) 43.
16. A. Jones, P. McAfee, R. Robinson, S. Zinreich and H. Wang, *J. Bone Joint Surg.* **70-A** (1988) 25.
17. M. Letts, T. Smallman, R. Afanasiev and G. Gouw, *J. Pediatric Orthop.* **6** (1986) 40.
18. P.C. McAfee, and H.A. Yuan, *Clin. Orthop.* **166** (1982) 62.
19. W. Meyerding, *Surg. Gynaecol. Obstet.* **54** (1932) 371.
20. F.L. Neugebauer, in *The New Sydenham Society Selected Monographs Vol.121*, trans F. Barnes, (The New Sydenham Society, London, 1888)
21. P.H. Newman, *J. Bone Joint Surg.* **45-B** (1963) 39.
22. R.O. Nicol, and J.H. Scott, *Spine* **11** (1986) 1027.
23. R.W. Porter, and W. Park, *J. Bone Joint Surg.* **64-B** (1982) 344.

24.   S. Seitsalo, K. Österman and M. Poussa, *Spine* **13** (1988) 899.
25.   A.D. Steffee, and Sitkowski, *Clin. Orthop.* **227** (1988) 82.
26.   R.H. Turner and A.J. Bianco, *J. Bone Joint Surg.* **53-A** (1981) 1298.
27.   L.L. Wiltse, J.G. Bateman, R.H. Hutchinson and W.E. Welson, *J. Bone Joint Surg.* **50-A** (1968) 919.
28.   L.L. Wiltse and D. Jackson, *Clin. Orthop.* **117** (1976) 92.

CHAPTER 11

ANKYLOSING SPONDYLITIS

A.C. Ross and M. Dolman

1. Introduction

Ankylosing spondylitis (AS) is a seronegative spondyloarthropathy of unknown aetiology. In common with other spondyloarthropathies there is involvement of the sacroiliac joints, insertional tendinitis, a peripheral arthropathy and an absence of rheumatoid factor in the serum. The disease is said to be primary if no other rheumatological disorder can be identified, or secondary if the sacroiliitis is caused by psoriatic arthropathy, Reiter's syndrome or inflammatory bowel disease. The diagnosis can be made if a patient complains of low back pain and a sacroiliitis is seen on a plain AP radiograph of the pelvis. Typically, patients are young men under the age of 40 years at presentation and give a history of back pain of insidious onset which has lasted for more than three months. Morning stiffness is common and pain is improved by regular exercise. The HLA B27 antigen is present in the serum of between 88 and 96% of patients with primary ankylosing spondylitis but in only 50% of those in whom the condition is secondary.

Ankylosing spondylitis is present in between 0.25 and 1% of the population but occurs forty times as frequently in relatives of those with the disease. Men are probably affected only two or three times as commonly as women although earlier work suggested that the ratio was much higher (10:1). The worldwide incidence exhibits wide geographical and racial variation. It is particularly common in Caucasians. HLA B27 is inherited as an autosomal co-dominant characteristic. Between 5 and 20% of those with the antigen develop ankylosing spondylitis. An environmental trigger appears to initiate the disease in susceptible individuals.

Pathologically, the spondyloarthropathies are distinct in affecting the enthesis, that is, the insertion of capsule and ligament into bone. Inflammatory change results not in the joint destruction and instability seen in rheumatoid arthritis but in progressive fibrosis, ossification and ankylosis. The sacroiliac joints are always involved but the tendon and ligamentous insertions onto the iliac crest, ischial tuberosities, greater trochanters, calcanei and patellae may also be affected.

2. Ankylosing spondylitis and the spine

In the spine, AS attacks the outer fibres of the annulus fibrosus at their line of insertion into the vertebral body. Granulation tissue grows into the intervertebral disc and is replaced by fibrous tissue which may subsequently ossify. Erosion of the anterior margins of the vertebral body causes a 'squaring off' of its normally concave shape on lateral radiographs. Progressive ossification of the annulus (syndesmophyte formation) and anterior longitudinal ligament result in the characteristic 'bamboo spine' appearance of late disease. In the posterior elements of the spine, there is a synovitis of the apophyseal joints with synovial hyperplasia and focal accumulation of lymphoid and plasma cells causing bone erosion, cartilage destruction, fibrosis and ankylosis. The macroscopic changes are reflected in the radiographic appearance of the spine.

3. Clinical assessment

Symptoms often start in the late teens and early twenties although the median age of onset has increased from 18 years in the decade 1930-40 to 28 years in 1981/2[2]. The median delay between the onset of symptoms and diagnosis has decreased but is still in the region of two years.

Typically, patients complain of low back pain, often with bilateral radiation to the knees which is worse in the morning, when it is accompanied by stiffness, and after rest. The pain is usually bilateral and is relieved by exercise. With increasing involvement of the spine, it is perceived as arising at progressively higher levels in the spine. As the costovertebral joints become involved, patients complain of pleuritic-type chest pain which is exacerbated by deep breathing and coughing.

In the small number of patients in whom spinal disease progresses relentlessly to complete bony ankylosis with deformity, pain becomes less and the symptoms of deformity predominate. There is a progressive loss of visual field which restricts outdoor activities and which may lead to profound depression. The patient may become pathologically preoccupied with his body image. Severe kyphotic deformity of the cervical spine can cause difficulty in eating and swallowing.

Slowly progressive sciatic pain in a patient with long-standing disease may occasionally be due to spinal stenosis but may, rarely, presage the onset of a full-blown cauda equina syndrome with bladder and bowel impairment.

In one-third of patients, back pain may be accompanied by an asymmetrical peripheral arthropathy which may precede the onset of spinal symptoms. They usually present with a monoarthritis of the hip or knee with minimal symptoms of pain or stiffness in the other large joints of the lower limbs. The upper limb joints are less frequently affected and involvement of the small joints of the hands and feet is rare. Enthesopathic symptoms may be present at any site of tendon, ligament or capsular insertion into bone.

4. Clinical signs

Sacroiliac joint tenderness may be elicited early in the disease by springing the pelvis in the prone, supine or lateral positions. This sign disappears if both sacroiliac joints are ankylosed. The earliest sign of lumbar spine involvement is a flattening of the lumbar lordosis followed by decreased flexibility in the sagittal and coronal planes. Paraspinal muscle spasm may be present. If the disease is allowed to progress, a fixed kyphosis may occur in the lumbar, thoracic or cervical spine. Chest expansion is classically diminished as a result of costovertebral joint involvement. If this is associated with a significant thoracic kyphosis, breathing becomes diaphragmatic and the vital capacity is markedly diminished. Jaw opening may be restricted by temporomandibular joint involvement or by abutment of the chin on the chest where there is a severe cervical kyphosis. Significant involvement of the hips causes stiffness and fixed flexion contractures which may be severe. Standing and walking are accompanied by voluntary flexion of the knees in order to compensate for the fixed flexion deformities in the hips and spine, and in order to improve the visual horizon. Fixed flexion of the knees may develop as a result of this or as a primary event.

5. Conservative management

The aim of conservative management is to control pain and stiffness and to minimise deformity.

Pain control is achieved using NSAIDs. The drug of choice currently is Indocid: second-line agents such as sulphasalazine may be used in resistant cases.

The importance of physiotherapy to maintain extension and reduce any flexion deformity must be emphasised to the patient. Patients should be encouraged to remain active and are given extension exercises to carry out at home at least twice each day. Attention should be paid to the maintenance of good posture, particularly at work. The recreational sport of choice is swimming. If the disease is aggressive, it may be necessary to admit the patient to a specialist rheumatology unit for pain control and exercises.

Radiotherapy has been used in the past to treat the spinal manifestations of ankylosing spondylitis. Its benefit was never dramatic and the risk of leukaemia is too great to warrant its continued usage.

6. Indications for surgery

There are no absolute indications for lumbar osteotomy. A significant number of patients with ankylosing spondylitis have fixed curves with minimal angulation which cause little disability or distress. These patients require support and reassurance but no surgical intervention.

At the other end of the scale, there are a small number of patients with severe curves which make it impossible for them to stand, sit or lie down in comfort. The loss of visual field may limit them to indoor activities and may significantly impair their capacity for both work and recreation. Because the kyphosis of ankylosing spondylitis develops over a prolonged period of time, many patients progressively adapt to the restrictions imposed by the deformity. For some, however, the progressive change in body image combined with increasing disability leads to a deterioration in self-esteem and clinical depression. It is those who do not adapt, and who have a significant deformity in the thoracic or lumbar spine without fixed deformity at the hips or knees, and in whom this condition causes significant distress or depression, who become candidates for a lumbar extension osteotomy. If a patient fulfils these criteria, is of an appropriate age and physical condition to undergo the procedure, and accepts the risks involved after a full explanation from the surgeon who will carry out the operation, then the operation may proceed.

7. Preoperative assessment

Preoperative assessment should be carried out jointly by a surgeon and anaesthetist who are skilled in the management of these problems. Specific anaesthetic problems are the need to have the patient in a prone position; rigidity and flexion of the cervical spine; temporomandibular joint involvement, which restricts mouth opening; fibrotic infiltration in the upper lobes may cause a functional pulmonary deficit with abnormal gas exchange; aortic valve incompetence and conduction defects increase with the duration of the disease from 3.5% after fifteen years to 10% at thirty years.

Specialised fibre-optic intubation techniques developed over the last twenty years have simplified the intubation of patients with rigid flexed necks and limited mouth opening but these can still prove difficult even in experienced hands, and ample time should be allowed for anaesthesia and positioning of the patient on the operating table.

8. Operative technique

There are three basic approaches to lumbar osteotomy which may be considered by reviewing their historical development.

8.1. Smith-Petersen lumbar extension osteotomy

The first lumbar osteotomy was carried out in March 1941 by Smith-Petersen although his formal description did not appear until 1945[14]. He described osteotomies in the lumbar spine at one or more levels to compensate for deformity in the thoracic spine. The spinous processes were cut into thin lamellae and excised at their bases. The ligamentum flavum was next detached from the inferior laminae and facets. The osteotomy was carried out obliquely through the facet joints at sufficient levels to allow adequate correction of the deformity. Closure was achieved by elevating the head and foot of the operating table. There was no suggestion that downward pressure on the osteotomy site was needed. After wound closure, the patient was kept in a plaster shell for four to six weeks and wore an extension brace for one year. It is clear from the cases he described that although osteotomies were undertaken at up to three levels, the main correction occurred at a single level.

Smith-Petersen emphasised that overcorrection was to be avoided since this caused problems when sitting. Patients who have a rigid neck and undergo sufficient lumbar correction to achieve a 0° chin-brow angle cannot look down to a desk, table or to a book on their knees without considerable discomfort.

There have been many minor variations of this technique published over the years[1,7,8,10,13]. All involve a similar anterior opening wedge osteotomy and most of the more recently reported series use posterior spinal instrumentation. These operations have not been uncomplicated. Mortality in the earlier series has been reported at up to 10% from mesenteric artery thrombosis and rupture of the aorta and its branches[8]. Neurological complications, whether from root or cauda equina compression have occurred in most large series. A proportion have been transient but some have been permanent. The source of the greatest controversy has been the tension placed on vascular structures anteriorly, which was highlighted by Weatherley, Jaffray and Terry[17]. This is directly proportional to the degree of opening of the osteotomy. The earliest series show single level corrections of 90 degrees whereas more recent series have reduced this by at least one half. We now aim to correct to no more than 30 degrees at a single level. The other techniques described below have aimed to avoid these complications.

8.2. Multiple level osteotomy with fixation

The concept of multiple level osteotomies with segmental fixation was introduced in 1979 by Puschel and Zielke[11] with the aim of reducing the complication rate from short acute-angle lumbar osteotomies. The osteotomies are fashioned in the manner described by Smith-Petersen but less bone is excised at each level. Between 5 and 7 mm of bone are removed in the lateral portion of the osteotomy. Fixation was initially achieved using Harrington rods but subsequently by a pedicle screw system[4]. Osteotomies were sited between T12 or L1 and L4 in order to maximise the corrective lever arm and to minimise the risk of nerve damage.

The overall mortality was reduced from 12% to 2.3% in a series of 177 patients[5]. Complications occurred in 22.6% of patients; most were transient and probably implant related. The average correction achieved per segment was $9.5°$. The average loss of correction was 15% at a mean of 27 months follow-up. No pseudoarthroses occurred and a 'harmonious lordosis' was achieved in the lumbar spine. Back pain was reduced from 85% preoperatively to 25% in the immediate postoperative period and thence to 8% at follow-up.

The loss of correction in the lower thoracic spine has led the authors to extend the correction up to T9 and down to S1. Until the results of this change are published it must be assumed that this will lead to an increase in pedicle screw-related complications since the number of screw sites has been doubled.

The effect of corrective surgery on the lives of these patients has recently been examined using modified Arthritis Impact Measurement Scales (mAIMS)[3]. These combine measures of mobility, activity, pain, dexterity, anxiety and depression. General health status was also examined. Substantial improvement was seen in virtually all activities, in the amount of pain suffered by the patient and in general health status. These results can be attributed chiefly to the correction of posture and reduction in pain levels. They should not be perceived as being related to this particular surgical technique but are probably indicative of the improvement achieved by all types of osteotomy.

8.3. Posterior closing wedge osteotomy

Concerns about the prevalence of vascular damage following opening wedge osteotomy have been voiced by Weatherley and his colleagues based on their experience with two older patients[17]. This led Jaffray to modify his technique to a closing wedge osteotomy[6]. This approach has also been advocated by Thomasen[16], Thiranont and Netrawichien[15], and van Royen and Slot[12]. Closing wedge osteotomy avoids lengthening the anterior column but shortens the middle column, unlike the opening wedge osteotomy which lengthens the anterior column, leaves the middle column essentially unchanged and shortens the posterior column. One wonders, however, whether they will at some stage encounter the dural buckling described by Lehmer and his colleagues in their series of 45 closing wedge osteotomies for post-traumatic and post-surgical kyphosis[9]. To date, there are still under forty cases of closing wedge osteotomies for ankylosing spondylitis reported in the literature with an average follow-up of two years.

The largest series has been reported by van Royen and Slot[12]. They describe an osteotomy which excises a V-shaped wedge measuring 5-7 cm at its base and which includes spinous processes, laminae, articular processes and part of the floor and the roof of the intervertebral foramen. After freeing the cauda equina and both L4 nerve roots, a further wedge is removed from the back of the vertebral body which contains the remains of the pedicles. They comment that this results in profuse haemorrhage. The lateral walls are crushed and the transverse processes are excised. Pedicle screws, which have been sited above and below the osteotomy, are then tightened onto pre-bent H-frame rods. Patients are treated postoperatively on a circoelectric bed and then have a TLSO fitted at two weeks.

They report no deaths in 22 patients, six dural tears, eight infections - two of which were deep and necessitated the removal of metalwork, two mechanical failures of fixation and one transient paresis and neuropraxia following insufficient removal of bone. The average loss of correction was 2.7 degrees.

8.4. Preferred technique

For the last six years we have used a modified Smith-Peterson osteotomy combined with Steffee (VSP) fixation. Our patients have been in the fifth decade of life with no objective signs of peripheral vascular disease. Any fixed flexion at the hips is corrected before lumbar osteotomy is considered. Preoperatively we obtain DEXA scans of the lumbar spine and have been surprised to find that most of our patients have a bone density which falls within normal limits. We restrict the maximal correction at any one level to 30 degrees to prevent over-lengthening of the anterior column. If greater correction is needed, osteotomies are carried out at two or more levels. The osteotomies are sited as low as possible in the lumbar spine in order to maximise the correction achieved. We plan to fix two levels above and two below the osteotomy and L4/5 is therefore the favoured level for a single wedge. Bleeding is minimal (under 500 ml) because the correction is carried out through the calcified disc space. We find that little pressure is required to close the osteotomy. The amount of correction obtained at each level in a two-level osteotomy can be controlled through the protruding shanks of the Steffee screws which are sited after the wedges have been cut but before osteotomy. Unlike the closing wedge osteotomy of van Royen and Slot[12] we fix every level to maximise the rigidity of the system. Patients are mobilised in a TLSO after six days and wear this until bony union is demonstrated by tomography. Most are able to discard the brace after twelve weeks. Loss of correction and screw pull-out have not been a problem and there have been no major complications to date.

9. References

1.   H. Briggs, S. Keats, P.T. Schlesinger, *J. Bone Joint Surg.* **29-A** (1947) 1075.
2.   A. Calin, J. Elswood, S. Rigg, and S.M. Skevington, *J. Rheumatol.* **15** (1988) 1234.
3.   H. Halm, P. Metz-Stavenhagen and K. Zielke, *Spine* **20** (1995) 1612.
4.   H.-J. Hehne and K. Zielke, *Orthop. Praxis* **23** (1987) 552.
5.   H.-J. Hehne, K. Zielke and H. Bohm, *Clin. Orthop.* **258** (1990) 49.
6.   D. Jaffray, V. Becker and S. Eisenstein, *Clin. Orthop.* **279** (1992) 122.
7.   E.H. La Chapelle, *J. Bone Joint Surg.* **28** (1946) 851.
8.   W.A. Law, *Clin. Orthop.* **66** (1969) 70.
9.   S.M. Lehmer, L. Keppler, R.S. Biscup, P. Enker, S.D. Miller and A.D. Steffee, *Spine* **19** (1994) 2060.
10. M.J. McMaster, *J. Bone Joint Surg.* **67-B** (1985) 204.
11. J. Puschel and K. Zielke, *Z. Orthop.* **120** (1982) 338.
12. B.J. van Royen and G.H. Slot, *J. Bone Joint Surg.* **77-B** (1995) 117.
13. E.H. Simmons, *Clin. Orthop.* **128** (1977) 65.
14. M.N. Smith-Peterson, C.B. Larson and S.E. Aufranc *J. Bone Joint Surg.* **27-A** (1945) 1.
15. N. Thiranont and P. Netrawichien, *Spine* **18** (1993) 2517.
16. E. Thomasen, *Clin. Orthop.* **194** (1985) 142.
17. C. Weatherley, D. Jaffray and A. Terry, *Spine* **13** (1988) 43.

CHAPTER 12

ISOLATED DISC RESORPTION

H.V. Crock and S. Matsuda

1. Introduction - historical survey

In 1911 Goldthwait[11] published a paper entitled, "The lumbosacral articulation. An explanation of many cases of 'lumbago', 'sciatica' and paraplegia". He drew attention to the wide variations that are found in anatomical specimens of the articular processes at the lumbosacral junction. He was the first to draw attention to the frequency of certain congenital anomalies of the spinal column such as sacralisation of the fifth lumbar vertebra and variations in the posterior articulations. He pointed to the possible connection between these abnormalities, together with protruding disc tissues, and sciatic pain.

In 1927, Professor Vittorio Putti[14] delivered the Lady Jones Lecture at the University of Liverpool on "New conceptions in the pathogenesis of sciatic pain". This was a scholarly dissertation which provided a basis for the understanding of cases of sciatica in which the cause was related to alterations in intervertebral articulations and foramina. Nearly 70 years later it still stands as a monument to sound clinical observation backed up by excellent anatomical studies and with the best radiological examinations, including stereograms, which were available to him at that time. The following quotation from this work is appended because of its historical importance in the evolution of the understanding of sciatica.

"Recent researches have shown that the intervertebral foramina are not all of the same size. The foramen between the fifth lumbar vertebra and the sacrum is always the smallest, that between the fourth and fifth vertebrae the next larger, and that between the fourth and third usually the next, although sometimes the second and third were about equal. Quite contrary to the size of the foramen or canal is the size of the nerve root enclosed. The fifth is always largest, the fourth next to the largest, and the third smaller as a rule, although sometimes the second and third roots were about equal in size. In other words, the fourth and fifth lumbar roots are predisposed, on anatomical grounds, to be affected more than any others by changes in the canals through which they pass. This fact has an important bearing on the pathology of sciatica, seeing that the fourth and fifth lumbar roots constitute a large part of the sciatic nerve. When, furthermore, it is considered that the fourth and fifth lumbar vertebrae, owing to their position in the spine, are the most exposed of all the vertebrae to compression and strain, and hence are the favourite site of arthritic processes, one can easily understand the frequency of sciatic pain. So much for the vertebral canal; but we must also consider its content, the funiculus. The most recent researches on this subject are those of Bonniot[1] and

Forestier[9]. The conclusions of these two writers may be summarised as follows: The fourth and fifth lumbar nerves are those possessing the longest funicular portion of all those which constitute the lumbosacral plexus - namely, those with the longest course through intervertebral foramina. The funicular portion of the nerve, unlike the intraspinal portion, does not lie within the arachnoid, but is only clothed by dura mater, and is not bathed in cerebrospinal fluid. Around the funiculus there is a very rich venous plexus, which is much influenced by mechanical conditions outside the funiculus. The absence of arachnoid, and therefore of a protective layer of fluid, exposes the funiculus to outside mechanical influences, such as do not affect the root, while the surrounding venous plexus puts it at the mercy of any congestion and stasis that may occur in the neighbourhood from many causes. The intervertebral foramen for all these reasons constitutes a critical region, or as Sicard has happily named it, "carrefour de la doleur" - *i.e.* the crossroads of neuralgia. Any condition which modifies in the slightest degree the contents, or the container, at once induces a painful reaction, which is referred distally to the sciatic nerve"[3].

In 1932, P.C. Williams[16] published a paper entitled, "Reduced lumbosacral joint space. Its relation to sciatic irritation". This paper was based on the analysis of 107 cases of sciatica which had been examined during 1931. In 85 of these patients, satisfactory AP and lateral X-rays of the lumbosacral junction were available though no oblique films had been taken. Of these, 80 patients (94%) showed pathological changes which Williams considered sufficient to cause sciatic irritation. Included in this paper is an illustration taken from Virchow in 1857 showing a pathological specimen of a cartilaginous tumour attached to disc and protruding into the neural canal. This is probably one of the earliest illustrations of a disc prolapse.

Among the 80 cases analysed, he listed 5 different factors causing sciatic irritation as depicted in Table 1. Of the 59 cases with narrowed lumbosacral discs, the average age at onset of symptoms was 30 years and Williams commented that these patients undoubtedly presented the greatest degree of invalidism.

Table 1. Factors listed by Williams as being causes of sciatic irritation.

Factors causing sciatic irritation	Total	Male	Female
Sacroiliac arthritis	3	1	2
Spondylolisthesis	2	1	1
Lumbosacral anomaly	1	1	0
Hypertrophic arthritis	15	11	4
Narrowed lumbosacral disc	59	35	24
TOTAL	80	49	31

When the history of medicine in the 20th century is reviewed, it will be clear that one brief contribution to the literature on sciatica came to exert an overwhelming influence on thought and practice relating to its treatment. The paper was published by Mixter and Barr[13] in 1934 in the New England Journal of Medicine under the title: "Rupture of the intervertebral disc with involvement of the spinal canal".

Professor Joseph Barr visited Australia in 1954, and delivered a lecture on disc prolapse as a cause of sciatica but warned against the dangers of its overzealous diagnosis and treatment. Regrettably his warning continues to go unheeded in 1996, more than 40 years later.

The last quarter of this present century has witnessed amazing developments in the fields of anaesthesia, imaging technologies and instrument design, each of which has profoundly influenced practices in spinal surgery. Sciatica is now treated by many different specialists ranging from neurologists, rheumatologists and psychiatrists to chiropractors, osteopaths and physiotherapists. Its surgical treatment rests largely with neurosurgeons and orthopaedic surgeons, the majority of whom perform only small numbers of spinal operations each year.

From the perspective of specialist spinal surgeons, it is clear that many people who treat patients with sciatica still have a simplistic view of disc disorders. They recognize only two entities - disc prolapse and disc degeneration. For them, removal of the disc prolapse may be attempted choosing a method from a bewildering array of techniques which includes open discectomy, micro discectomy, percutaneous discectomy, laser discectomy and intradiscal injections of discolytic agents such as chymopapain and chymodiactin.

Should the diagnosis be that of disc degeneration, they usually adopt one of the following 3 approaches:

i) Disc degeneration is regarded as an ageing process, the symptoms of which are to be expected and tolerated. Surgery is thought not to be indicated and the patients are referred for conservative management.

ii) Disc degeneration is believed to cause vertebral instability which produces pain and hence should be treated by spinal stabilisation. Methods include spinal fusion with or without fixation devices or spinal stabilisation without spinal fusion.

iii) Disc degeneration may give rise to spinal stenosis for which some form of spinal canal decompression can be performed, with or without spinal fusion, with or without internal fixation.

In a paper entitled "A reappraisal of intervertebral disc lesions", Crock[2] drew attention to a number of other disc disorders including internal disc disruption and isolated disc resorption of which the latter is the subject of the present chapter.

2. Isolated lumbar disc resorption

The terminology isolated disc resorption was coined by Crock in 1970, though he was unaware of the existence of William's paper[16] at that time. This condition is characterised by gross narrowing of one affected disc space with sclerosis of the adjacent vertebral bodies. Occurring commonly as an isolated finding in an otherwise normal spine, even late in life, it is seen most commonly at L5/S1, occasionally at L4/5 and rarely at higher levels in the lumbar spine (Figure 1). It causes back and leg pain more commonly than does prolapse of an intervertebral disc and therefore warrants identification as a specific form of disc disease.

3. Clinical presentations

Patients presenting with symptoms attributable to isolated disc resorption fall into 3 readily recognizable groups.

Group 1: Patients present with recurring attacks of severe back pain with buttock pain, which is usually bilateral. Attacks last for only a few days. In some patients an acute lumbar scoliosis will develop sometimes resulting in a tilt to one or other side of the midline, alternating during different attacks from left to right. These attacks may be

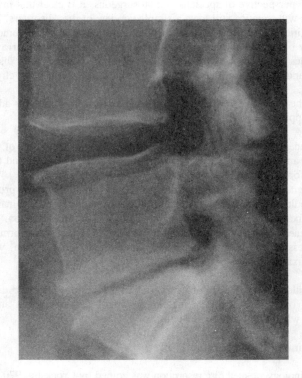

Figure 1. A lateral X-ray showing advanced isolated disc resorption at L5/S1 in a female patient aged 39 years.

shortlived. They are usually due to disc resorption above the lumbosacral junction or at the first mobile segment above a segmentation anomaly. Attacks usually come on without apparent cause. Recurring attacks may be separated by years.

Group 2: Acute back pain with unilateral sciatica coming on sometimes after a specific episode of trauma such as a fall on the buttocks or after a lifting episode occurring against a background of previous shortlived attacks as described above. These patients may be found to have an associated disc prolapse consisting largely of sequestrated vertebral endplate cartilage.

Following trauma, particularly a fall onto the buttocks, the symptoms may extend to include severe bilateral buttock and leg pains. In some cases, buttock and leg pain may be aggravated by standing or sitting and occasionally by walking. The description of nerve root claudication may then be used to describe this particular symptom pattern. Characteristically the leg pain is often relieved by postural changes such as stooping to bend forwards or after lying on a bed for a short time. Neurological examination is usually normal in these patients even when symptoms of referred leg pain are severe.

Group 3: Patients present eventually with intractable back pain, troublesome even at night, sometimes associated with referred buttock pain. When the L3/4 or L4/5 discs are affected, back pain often predominates and may be very severe, preventing any movement during attacks. Muscle spasm leads to lumbar tilt, a scoliotic deformity which may persist for hours, days or weeks at a time.

The clinical significance of isolated disc resorption is regrettably still not widely appreciated for a number of reasons. The first is that it is regarded by many as an innocuous form of degenerative disease of the spine which is often asymptomatic. While it may give rise to only trivial complaints in the majority of those who are found to have it, it is a potent cause of severe disability in a small percentage of patients. Many of these may be denied treatment because they present with symptoms only. Even when their pain is at its worst, they may have no abnormal neurological findings. The historical account of symptoms is often of more relevance in reaching a surgical decision about treatment than are the physical signs which can be elicited on clinical examination. Where MRI examinations are not available, radiculography is still used in investigating these patients. Almost invariably, the radiculograms are reported as normal and on this basis surgical treatment is frequently denied. Facet subluxation and ligamentum flavum buckling both contribute to venous obstruction in the intervertebral foramina and nerve root canals on either side of the resorbed disc space. This obstructive process interferes with venous drainage of the nerve roots which as a result become oedematous, a finding easily overlooked on the radiculograms[4,5,6,7].

4. Venous obstruction in the nerve root canals and intervertebral foramina

While the mechanical obstructions to the S1 nerve root in its canal and of the L5 nerve root in the adjacent foramen can be readily appreciated in cases of isolated disc resorption, the importance of the concomitant perineural venous obstruction is less widely recognised. The occlusion of veins that is found in advanced cases is the underlying cause of the deep-seated buttock and thigh pain which comes on after standing or sitting.

5. Imaging studies

5.1. *Plain X-rays*

This condition can be diagnosed initially using plain X-rays. Narrowing of a single lumbar intervertebral disc space usually develops over a number of years, the clinical course being punctuated by repeated bouts of acute low back pain lasting 3-4 days which then resolve completely. In the lower lumbar region in adults, the disc height between adjacent vertebral end plates ranges from 10-15 mm. In established cases of isolated lumbar disc resorption, the height of the intervertebral disc space may be reduced to 3 mm. The vacuum phenomenon of Knuttson (black gas shadow in the disc space) is another prominent radiological feature, especially in X-rays taken with the patient standing with the lumbar spine extended. Sclerosis of the adjacent vertebral end plates appears and often extends to involve large areas of the vertebral bodies (Figure 2). Marginal osteophyte formation is often minimal but a ridge of bone covered with a thin layer of annular fibre

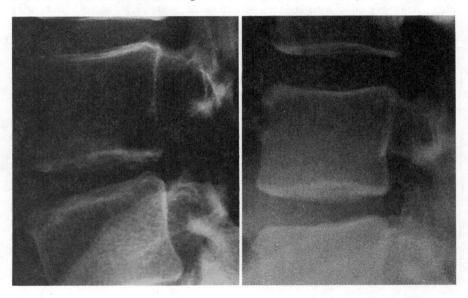

Figure 2. (a) A lateral radiograph showing an early isolated disc resorption at L4/5 with loss of disc height of the order of 50% and a sclerosis in the vertebral end plates. (b) An X-ray of the same disc space taken 3 ½ years later showing extensive sclerosis in the anterior two thirds of the vertebral body of L4 extending upwards by about a third of the height of the vertebral body. This type of change is associated with punctate lesions in the end plates similar to those shown in Figure 6

remnants frequently projects into the spinal canal across its whole width. Subluxation of the facet joints related to the resorbed disc is an invariable finding best seen in oblique views of the facets (Figure 3). Retrolisthesis of L5 on S1 may occur, further compromising the sizes of the nerve root canals and intervertebral foramina.

The disc space narrowing which accompanies sacralisation anomalies should not be confused with that occurring in isolated lumbar disc resorption (Figure 4). However, disc resorption at the first mobile segment above a sacralised vertebra is common. Disabling symptoms may occur as a result and sciatic scoliosis is commonly seen. Symptoms of bilateral buttock and leg pain may become intractable in established cases, the leg pains usually radiating down the backs of the thighs towards the knee joints.

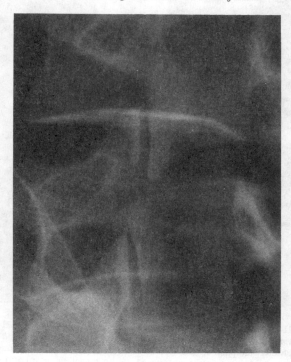

Figure 3. An oblique view of the lumbar spine of a 43 year old male showing S1 facet intrusion at L5/S1. Note the apex of the S1 facet lying in close proximity to the inferior margin of the pedicle of L5.

5.2. MRI and CT

The basic pathology of isolated disc resorption is still incompletely understood. It appears that there are active biochemical processes leading to degradation of the nuclear and annular portions of the intervertebral disc and eventually to necrosis of the vertebral endplate cartilages. When vertebral endplate sclerosis extends into the vertebral body, seen best in magnetic resonance imaging, but even on plain X-rays, this condition may be mistaken for an infective or neoplastic process in the vertebral bodies, Sauser *et al*[15]., Demos[8], Miskew *et al.*[12] (Figure 5).

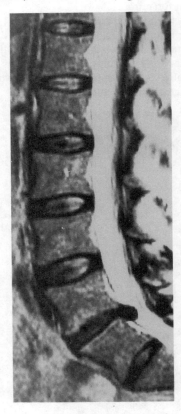 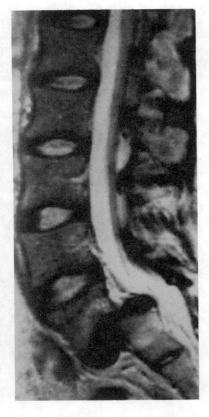

Figure 4. MRI of the lumbar spine (T2 weighted sequence) showing a mid-sagittal section in a 55 year old female with disc resorption at L5/L6 above a segmentation anomaly. There is a large sequestrated fragment of disc projecting into the spinal canal. Note the signal changes in the vertebral end plates on either side of the disc from which the nuclear signal is lost.

Figure 5. T2 weighted MRI of the lumbar spine of a 38 year old female, mid-sagittal view, showing advanced isolated disc resorption at the site of a spondylolisthesis at L5/S1 with marked changes in signal in the vertebral bodies on either side of the disc space.

In some cases, the disc space narrowing is associated with punctate defects in opposing vertebral end plates. These lesions are best seen in horizontal CT images. MRI examination in these cases usually shows extensive changes in the vertebral bodies on either side of the end plates often involving half of each vertebra. Patients with this less common form of isolated disc resorption are often subjected to a wide variety of tests including vertebral biopsy (Figure 6).

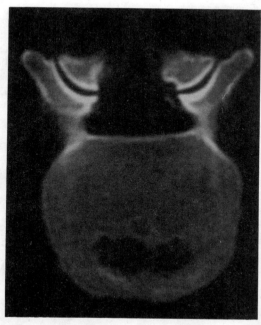

Figure 6. An axial CT image showing the punctate lesions which have developed in the vertebral end plate of L4 in a female patient aged 53 years. Note the early ossification visible in the ligamentum flavum on the right side of the image.

6. Treatment

Group 1: Most patients in group 1 will respond to conservative measures of treatment such as those practised by physical therapists. Bearing in mind that venous obstruction in the nerve root canals and intervertebral foramina is the principal underlying cause of the referred leg pain in these patients, prescription of low dose aspirin, in the form of Dispirin CV 100 mg daily or soluble aspirin 75 mg one daily, will enhance the microcirculation in the region of the nerve root canals and intervertebral foramina, leading to rapid resolution of the referred leg pain.

Surgical treatment may be indicated for frequently recurring symptoms. Bilateral foraminal and nerve root canal decompressions, with preservation of the spinous processes and reattachment of the lumbodorsal aponeurosis to the midline supraspinous and interspinous ligaments at the end of the decompression procedure, will usually produce very satisfactory results.

Group 2: In patients who have unilateral sciatica which is unrelieved by conservative measures, the appropriate treatment is disc fragment excision and bilateral foraminal and nerve root canal decompressions.

During the evolution of this disorder, a number of patients may present with unilateral sciatica. They may exhibit classic features of neurological defects in either or both L5 and S1 roots. Usually there is a sequestrated fragment of vertebral endplate cartilage impinging on the affected nerve roots. At operation the disc space is virtually empty and clearly recognisable necrotic vertebral endplate cartilage will be found causing the nerve root compression. The volume of sequestrated material is often large. Clearance of resorbed retained fragments from within the disc space must be carried out with great care. Only fine rongeurs can be used and there is danger of these instruments penetrating anterior annular fibres and damaging intra-abdominal contents or great vessels such as the abdominal aorta, the vena cava or its tributaries (Figure 7).

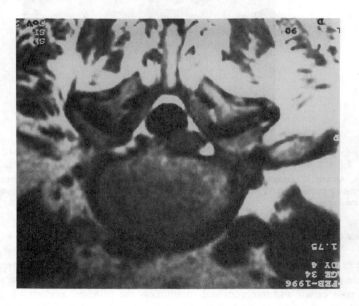

Figure 7. An axial view from the MRI study in Figure 4, showing a large, right-sided disc protrusion. The image is orientated in the position in which the patient would be lying on the operating table.

Group 3: In the group of patients with intractable back pain most commonly involving the L4/5 disc space, anterior interbody fusion can be recommended (Figure 8).

Detailed descriptions of the surgical techniques recommended for all of these groups have been published by Crock[6].

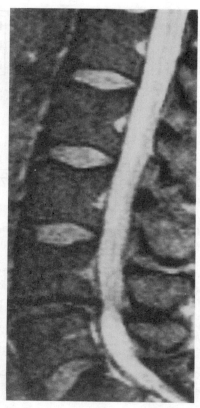

Figure 8. A T2-weighted MRI image of the lumbar spine of a 47 year old male patient with advanced isolated disc resorption at L4/5 showing the typical features of loss of nuclear signal, decrease in the height of the intervertebral disc and profound changes in the vertebral endplates. There is an associated canal stenosis at L4/5.

7. Current trends in management

Between 1992 and 1994 in a series of more than 400 spinal operations, we operated on 66 cases of isolated disc resorption. There were 47 cases at L5/S1 of which only 2 were treated by anterior interbody fusion. At L4/5 there were 16 cases of whom 4 were treated by anterior interbody fusion. At L3/4 there were three cases, one of which was treated by anterior interbody fusion (Figure 9). All others were treated by bilateral foraminal and nerve root canal decompressions.

Within the past three years, however, a variety of new techniques have been applied to the treatment of this disorder including interbody fusion using metallic cages inserted

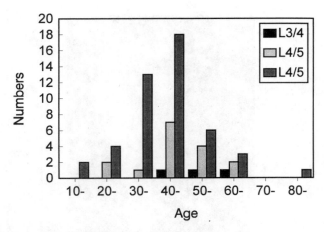

Figure 9. Age distribution of isolated disc resorption in the lumbar region. Data are from a consecutive series of 66 patients treated surgically between 1992-1994.

either retroperitoneally or with laparoscopic techniques and vertebral stabilisation without fusion using pedicle screws and elasticized bands, the Graf stabilisation technique. None of these methods can be recommended at present as satisfactory outcome studies have not been published[2].

8. Surgical outcome

In 1981, Venner and Crock[17] reported results of clinical studies of isolated disc resorption in the lumbar spine with good results in more than 70% of patients (Table 2).

Table 2. Success rate of the operation for isolated disc resorption in 45 patients based on six criteria

Criteria	Success rate, %
Operation considered by the patients to be "worthwhile"	84
Functional disability reduced	71
Return to work	78
Relief of backache	84
Relief of pain in the legs	91
Independent observer's assessment: Dr R M Venner, Good in	71

The overall success rate of the operation could be classified as follows:

Complete success (satisfying all 6 criteria)	62%
Partial success (3-5 criteria)	24%
Failure (< 3 criteria)	14%

In the 16 years following that publication, we have made a number of other important observations. The first is that in treating this lesion, when it is causing back pain and bilateral sciatica, the pathology should be modified by the surgery without any attempt to recreate normality in the spine[10]. There has been a move away from this principle in favour of a variety of methods of internal fixation associated with the use of pedicle screws or with anterior interbody fusion designed to recreate spinal normality by restoring intervertebral height and using both internal fixation devices anteriorly and posteriorly at the same time. These procedures are not required in most cases as excellent results can be achieved using the long established methods of foraminal and nerve root canal decompression which ensure satisfactory perineural venous refilling and relieve referred leg pains. Where spinal fusion is indicated, it is most safely performed by anterior interbody fusion performed extraperitoneally under direct division. The use of laparoscopic methods will doubtless evolve but at present they are time-consuming and potentially dangerous, as the great vessels on the posterior abdominal wall are often adherent to the surface of the disc in advanced cases of isolated disc resorption, particularly at the L4/5 level.

Another observation of great importance concerns the secondary changes which may occur above the level of an isolated disc resorption even when the disc space at that level remains of normal height. Laminal and facet hypertrophy may produce secondary stenoses which again respond satisfactorily to conservative foraminal and nerve root canal decompressions.

The final observation applies to patients with quite large disc prolapses producing sciatica without limitation of straight leg raising or loss of limb reflexes. In these cases, conservative treatment with low dose aspirin and graduated exercise based on walking alone, will often result in relief of the sciatica. On review with MRI after a period of 9-12 months the disc prolapse may have spontaneously resorbed. This process of autodigestion is a feature of disc resorption but its mechanism is still incompletely understood.

Looking back to the observations made by Goldthwait, Williams, Putti and others in the early years of this century, it is amazing to note how close they came to recognising some of the causes of sciatic pain relating to changes in the intervertebral foramina and affecting the perineural venous drainage of lumbar nerve roots. Even today, the attention of many specialists remains focused on the entity of disc prolapse. When isolated disc resorption is confused with disc prolapse, the outcome for patients is often poor. Disc excision alone will fail to relieve their leg pain. Multiple operations may follow, sometimes involving 3 or 4 lumbar intervertebral levels, with disastrous consequences for the patient and family concerned.

9. Summary

Isolated disc resorption is a condition found commonly on X-ray. Most cases respond to conservative treatment. Some will require surgical treatment in the form of bilateral foraminal and nerve root canal decompressions. Occasionally interbody fusion may be required. Internal fixation devices should not be used.

10. References

1.   A. Bonniot. Anatomie du plexus lombaire chez l'homme. *Arch. de Morphol* (1922) 12.

2.   H.V. Crock. *Med. J. Aust.* **1** (1970) 983-989.

3.   H.V. Crock. *J. Bone Joint Surg.* **63B** (1981) 487-490.

4.   H.V. Crock. *Clin. Orthop.* **115** (1976) 109-115.

5.   H.V. Crock, M. C. Crock. *Neuro-Orthopaedics* **5** (1988) 96-99.

6.   H. V. Crock. *A Short Practice of Spinal Surgery*. Second Edition (Springer-Verlag, Wien, New York, 1993).

7.   H.V. Crock, in The Lumbar Spine and Back Pain, 4th edn., ed. M.I.V. Jayson, (Churchill Livingstone, 1992) 307-312.

8.   T. C. Demos. *Orthopaedics* **4** (1981) 77-79.

9.   H. Forestier. La sciatique d'origine sacro-vertebrale. *Bull. et Mem. de la Soc. de Med. de Paris* **28** (1914).

10.   P. Gallinaro, E. Indemini, G. Tabasso, G. Massazza, Stenosi del canale radiculare da degenerazione discale. Stenosis of the nerve root canal caused by disc resorption, *Chir. Organi. Mov.* **LXXVII** (1992) 61-63.

11.   J. E. Goldthwait. The lumbosacral articulation. An explanation of many cases of "lumbago", "sciatica" and "paraplegia". *Boston Med. and Surg. J.* **CLXIV No. 11** (1911) 365-372.

12.   D. Miskew, J. McClellan, J. Rodriguez. *Spine* **6** (1981) 39-42.

13.   W. J. Mixter, J. S. Barr. *New Engl. J. Med.* **211** (1934) 210-215.

14.   V. Putti. Lady Jones Lecture on New conceptions in the pathogenesis of sciatic pain. Lancet **2** (1927) 53-60.

15.   D. Sauser, A.B. Goldman, J. J. Kaye. Journal de l'Association Canadienne des Radiologistes **29** (1978) 44-50.

16.   P. C. Williams. JAMA **99** (1932) 1677-1682.

17.   R.M. Venner, H.V. Crock. *J. Bone Joint Surg.* **63B** (1981) 491-494.

CHAPTER 13

POSTERIOR LUMBAR INTERBODY FUSION AND CAGES

M.R.K. Karpinski

1. Introduction

The concept of spinal fusion originated in the early part of the 19th Century as a stabilising procedure for spondylitic progressive post-poliomyelitic and tuberculous spinal deformity[1,28,29,35]. An expansion of the indications for this procedure then followed. The hypothesis was simple: immobilisation of the functional spinal unit would eliminate or reduce pain by preventing irritative factors acting on the intervertebral disc, facet joints and other pain sensitive structures. As a consequence a variety of fusion techniques evolved; anterior[15,53,58], posterior, postero-lateral[45], posterior lumbar interbody fusion (PLIF)[10,11,23] and Global Circumferential Fusions[24]. Each technique, with its associated proponent, claimed benefits, disadvantages and complications. A repeating theme became apparent: the correlation of a successful arthrodesis of the spine and relief of symptoms was obscure[16,52] and unpredictable[17].

In a meta-analysis of lumbar spine fusion techniques, the PLIF gave both the highest satisfactory clinical outcome and fusion rates[60]. Historically Mercer[41], in 1936, is credited with the first use of the interbody fusion for spondylolisthesis, whilst Jaslow[31] (1946) reported the PLIF after lumbar discectomy. Undoubtedly the father and pioneer of this technique was Cloward[10,11]. At meetings he has claimed that the origins of this disc substitution by bone came about from the Pearl Harbour bombings in 1941, in which young U.S. Marines ruptured their intervertebral discs and on seeking treatment, posed the question "what replaced the disc?". Hence the PLIF was born.

However, its popularity dwindled. The operation was technically demanding with a steep learning curve and a high potential for complications. A gradual resurgence of interest followed[38,65], culminating in the first symposium on the PLIF chaired by Lin in 1985 and the Proceedings were published in Clinical Orthopaedics and Related Research Volume 193. History repeated itself as many surgeons were unable to reproduce the good results and popularity for this technique again fell. In order to achieve a higher clinical and biological success, a number of aids were developed. Pedicular screw and plate fixation systems[18], carbon fibre implants6,7 and fusion cages[2,48,49].

2. Indications

A tabulated form of proposed indications appears in Table 1. The plethora of indications for the PLIF suggests a boot looking for a foot to fit and it is worth examining these indications further.

Table 1. Indications for Posterior Lumbar Interbody Fusion

1.	Discogenic low back pain.
2.	Spondylolysis
3.	Grade I and II spondylolisthesis
4.	Recurrent disc herniation.
5.	Failed chemonucleolysis
6.	Spinal stenosis

2.1. Discogenic Low Back Pain

This is a diffuse term often defying pain source identification; it is estimated that less than 10% of low back pain aetiology is diagnosed correctly. Both the intervertebral disc and posterior longitudinal ligaments are innervated[5,26,34,46,51], and provocative discography may help to assess a patient's suitability for fusion[55]. However, the complex multi-level innervation of the functional spinal unit leads to difficulty in interpreting the pain source and the fact that a normal disc can be rendered symptomatic complicates the matter further[43]. The efficacy of discography therefore remains unresolved. Proponents consider the technique essential[62] whilst others are unimpressed by the ability to predict successful lumbar spine fusions for low back pain[12,43].

The concept and role of 'lumbar instability' in discogenic low back pain is ill-conceived, poorly understood and lacks reproducible clinical and radiological data[42]. With the advent of MRI, greater detail and understanding in the staging of disc degeneration is possible and there now exists some correlation between the images of severe disc degeneration and symptomatic changes[59].

In spite of provocative dynamic and static investigations, patient selection for fusion remains at least in part an 'art form'. Naylor[44] proposed an elegant theory for the biochemical and biophysical aetiology of disc degeneration and pain production. This lends itself to the hypothesis that the excision of the posteriorly innervated discal structures and the total or subtotal nucleotomy with a successful PLIF would not only provide rigidity and abolish a mechanical pain stimulus but would eradicate any biochemical source of pain factors. Posterior fusions alone do not abolish all functional spinal unit movement[50] and anterior interbody fusions do not address the posterior discal nociceptors[22].

2.2. Spondylolysis and Spondylolisthesis

Spinal fusion for spondylolysis and spondylolisthesis is performed on the assumption that the spondylolytic lesion is the origin of 'Back Pain'. Fusion techniques, with or without instrumentation, are usually successful. There remains, however, a subgroup of patients with high degree, long-standing slips and symptomatic degeneration of discs above and below the lysis which may not respond satisfactorily. In this group of patients, an interbody fusion, cage with or without instrumentation, may be indicated[3], Figure 1.

2.3. Failed Back Syndrome

This term encompasses conditions such as recurrent disc herniation, arachnoiditis and

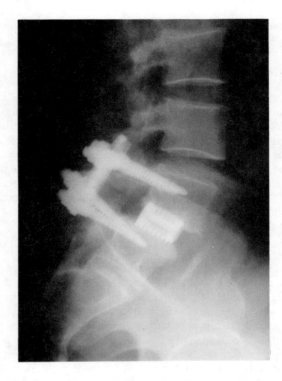

Figure 1. 18 months post-operative radiographs from a 28 year old male following relocation of Grade II spondylolisthesis treated with a Stryker 2S pedicular screw and plate system and a ray interbody fusion cage.

peri-neural fibrosis following previous back surgery. The goal of the interbody fusion is to prevent further disc herniations and stiffen the functional spinal unit in an attempt to eliminate or reduce the mechanical stimulation of scar production and neural irritation. Secondary, tertiary and further procedures carry increasingly limited benefits.

2.4. Failed chemonucleolysis

Chemonucleolysis is a proven efficacious alternative to open discectomy, being successful in alleviating sciatic symptoms in 75% of carefully selected patients. Persistent post-injection back pain is unusual and attributable to a non-specific inflammatory reaction[33]. It is proposed that these chemonucleolysis failures be treated by posterior lumbar interbody fusion[55].

3. Surgical procedure

The posterior approach to the lumbar sacral spine and the intervertebral disc is fundamentally the same for both the PLIF and interbody fusion cages.

3.1. Technique

Under general hypotensive anaesthesia, the abdomen free of compression and with radiological confirmation of the level, posterior spinal elements are approached, preserving the supraspinous and interspinous ligaments. Fenestrotomies are carried out bilaterally with partial medial facetectomies. The degree of facet and ligament excision is dictated by need for space and the type or configuration of bone graft or cage to be used. The appropriate intervertebral disc is identified and, after retraction and protection of both the exiting and medial nerve roots, the disc is excised and the space preparation proceeds. This may be performed piecemeal or using special graduated instrumentation, *ie.* box chisels, drills, corers[10,11,40]. A total or subtotal nuclear discectomy is performed to inhibit soft tissue invasion of the grafted disc space[25]. Detailed operative procedures can be obtained from the original articles.

3.2. Grafting

Autografts are quicker to incorporate than other grafts; allografts are also successful and have the advantage of availability, size, shape and quantity with no additional surgery for harvesting[9,21]. The whole intervertebral disc may be replaced by bone using tricortico-cancellous bone or the Unipour concept[38]. In dowel techniques[4,65], the graft should be positioned laterally as this is better biomechanically[20]. The ideal role of the graft is to provide immediate post-operative stability leading on to osseous integration. It is known that grafts are weakened mechanically during the phase of creeping substitution, and may collapse and resorb during this phase. A keystone graft construction is superior to a Cloward configuration with respect to the surface area available for fusion and graft extrusion and collapse[56,64].

The introduction of carbon cages [6,7], has enhanced a quicker and more reliable fusion experimentally with encouraging early clinical results. Hydroxyapatite interbody grafts are stiffer and lessen disc height loss[14]. Augmentation of interbody fusion has recently mushroomed with the development of multiple cage-type implants (*eg.* Stryker, BAK, TFC). These must not detract from the basic principle that the objective is to obtain an interbody fusion. The implant acts as a vehicle for the bone graft, helping to prevent collapse and extrusion and maintaining disc height.

4. Advantages and disadvantages

Interbody fusion is biomechanically advantageous compared with other techniques, it has a higher rate of fusion (94.5%) and the best clinically satisfactory results (74.5%)[61]. It can be performed as a floating fusion with reduced iatrogenic morbidity to adjacent functional spinal units, although some experimental observation has shown increased motion at the adjacent segments[47]. The clinical relevance at this point is uncertain[37]. The necessity and efficacy of distraction is questionable. Successful fusion with a graft collapse and graft *in situ* by open and percutaneous methods are well recognised[32,57]. Nerve root canals can be decompressed simultaneously at surgery without the need for major distraction which carries the potential for complications and neuropathological changes[8,39]. The claims for restoration of spinal alignment infers a major deformity and the term would be better replaced; graft collapses and disc height decreases cannot be synonymous with re-alignment. Newer interbody implants incorporate features to restore lumbar lordosis. The inhibition of post-operative adhesion formation is theoretical and at present confirmatory studies are awaited.

The main disadvantage of the PLIF is a slow learning curve and potentially serious complications and these have resulted in the PLIF remaining out of favour for many years. It is technically demanding and, initially, single level operations can take three to four hours, reducing to two hours as experience is gained.

Complications of nerve root injury, both transient and permanent, with graft extrusion are the most common. Surprisingly little published data exists on these. Taking an aggregate of published series, the instance of these complications is less than 1% for dural tears, leaks, graft resorption, collapse and neurological complications[13,40]. These may be misleadingly low in that the authors of both of these series are very experienced surgeons.

5. Interbody fusion cages

Interbody fusion cages have been designed to separate the implant and biological functions of the PLIF[6,7]. The implant fulfills the mechanical needs of the PLIF whilst acting as a conduit for the bone graft for biological union. There are many designs, and specifications can be obtained from the appropriate commercial source. Using one should not detract from the aim and fundamental concept of the PLIF.

The instrumented cage is user friendly and the natural extrapolation from discectomy to implant, using precision instrumentation, is simple. The availability of multiple sizes of implants obviates the need for harvesting of iliac bone and its recognised complications. With the tide of enthusiasm however, the surgeon must anticipate the potential complications of implant failure, loosening, migration and infection.

Before embarking on this type of surgery questions should be asked about what measures would avoid these complications. Can the implant be removed safely and what salvage procedure would exist? The author is an enthusiast for the PLIF and has undertaken two pilot studies using
    a) the Ray threaded fusion cage
    b) Stryker Ogival cage.

5.1. Threaded Fusion Cages
The Ray Fusion Cages[48, 49] are thin walled threaded tubular shells of titanium with large, 1.5 x 4 mm, perforations. The cage shell is about 70% perforated on the superior and inferior sides. The sides are blocked to prevent potential ingrowth. The cages are supplied in sizes 14, 16 or 18 mm outside diameter. They are designed to be inserted both posteriorly and anteriorly. The intervertebral disc is drilled, threaded bilaterally using a

tap, and paired cages are introduced. Bone graft, approximately 5 cm³, is impacted into the hollow shell and the cages are closed by a plastic cover. The cage provides immediate fixation and prevents retrograde expulsion of the bone graft.

The early results from threaded fusion cages in 6 males and 12 females, average age 44 years (range 32-49) are promising. The indications were discogenic low back pain in 13, failed back surgery 4 and one case of spondylolisthesis grade II. The spinal levels affected were 4 at L4/5, 10 at L5/S1 and 4 at both of these. After a minimum follow-up of 9 months (maximum 21 months) the functional outcome was

Good	Patients symptomatically and markedly improved. Back to work, domestic and recreational chores. No significant disability	10
Improved	Patient back to work. Some restriction of recreational and domestic activities. Occasional analgesics.	4
Same	Pain and disability continues requiring analgesics, conservative treatment.	2
No better/ worse	Deterioration, further restriction in work and social/recreational activities. Regular analgesics.	2

The functional outcome of this cohort of patients is constantly under review and the final outcome will be judged independently. Two patients had complications of a transient L5 nerve root palsy and neuropraxia which fully resolved. There has been no evidence of metal failure, retrograde expulsion, aseptic or septic loosening in any of the cages.

It has not been possible from plain radiographs to detect bone continuity between the upper and lower vertebral bodies. Flexion/extension radiographs have been performed on some patients which confirm absence of movement at the caged functional spinal unit. It has been impossible to differentiate whether complete stiffness has occurred at the vertebral endplate interfaces with the cage or whether bone graft has grown through the cavities in the implant and integrated with the vertebral body above and below.

Five patients have been subjected to MRI scanning, (Figures 2 and 3). Images have been compromised by artefact formation, where the cage has been well visualised and the continuity of bone graft cannot be identified with certainty. One patient required re-operation for faulty positioning of the TFC with L5 nerve root involvement. At re-operation two weeks after the initial procedure, there was some resistance to removal of the cage and inspection of the inner contents revealed that the bone graft had become an amalgam with offshoots through the fenestrations in the outer shell.

5.2. Stryker Ogival Cage

The Stryker Ogival cage (Figure 4) is made of titanium coated with 60 μm thick layer of Hydroxylapatite. It is open on four sides, bullet shaped anteriorly and closed posteriorly with a thread to facilitate introduction. It comes in four sizes: 9, 10, 11 and 12 mm in height and 25 mm in length. The large diameter is 13, 14, 15 and 16 mm respectively. The

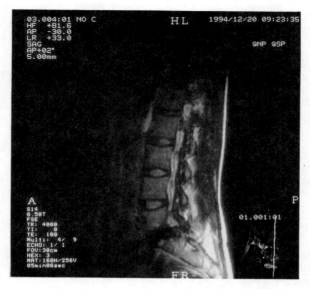

Figure 2. Post-operative MRI scan of 34 year old female showing artifacts at L5/S1 level. The functional result was excellent and pain free at 15 months.

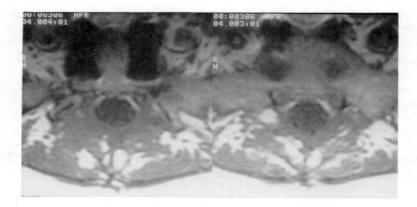

Figure 3. Transverse MR images at L5/S1 of Ray threaded fusion cage showing some artifact. There is very little gadolinium enhanced material intra-spinally. This was functionally a good result.

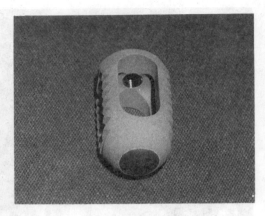

Figure 4. Stryker hydroxylapatite-coated Ogival interbody fusion cage.

superior window is 6.5 mm wide and the lateral windows are sequentially 4, 5, 6 and 7 mm in width.

The cage is inserted through a posterior approach using specialised instruments after preparation of a disc by drilling and reaming the space only. The size of the implanted cage corresponds to the size of the reamer which fits tightly in the intervertebral disc space. The corresponding Ogival cage is packed with either autogenous or allograft bone and impacted into the prepared space relying on its stability by press fit and secondly by fine ridges on its superior and inferior surfaces, analogous to a barbed hook which prevents retrograde expulsion.

Thirty three patients, 18 males and 15 females, with a mean age of 39 years (range 28-63) had a fusion peformed using a Styker Ogival fusion cage. The indications were discogenic low back pain in 22 cases, failed back surgery in 9 cases and 2 cases of spondylolisthesis. The maximum follow-up at the time of writing is six months. The levels affected were 9 at L4/5, 19 at L5/S1 and 5 at both of these. There are no apparent complications and no failures associated with the implant, retrograde expulsion, aseptic or septic loosening. At present the study is in its infancy and full functional results are therefore unavailable. The longterm assessment of patients will be carried out by an independant observer. The initial clinical impression is favourable. Patients are subjected to per-operative, post-operative three, six and 12 monthly follow up check x-rays. The follow up x-rays show well visualised intra-cage bone graft. Three patients have undergone MRI Scanning which produced artifact. One patient has had a CT scan which showed evidence of bony continuity in the transverse plane (Fig 5).

6. Discussion

The concept and philosophy of the posterior lumbar interbody fusion is biomechanically correct in the way it addresses the discogenic 'problem' and in

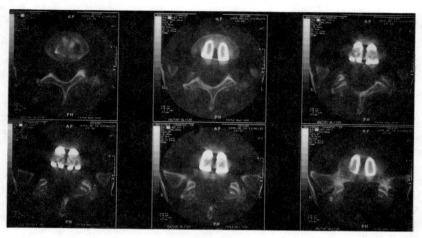

Figure 5. CT scan of L5/S1 showing the Ogival interbody fusion cage in a 34 year-old male. There is evidence of bony continuity transversely.

experienced hands carries the best results for spinal fusion both clinically and radiologically. However, it is disadvantaged by potentially serious per-operative complications: graft collapses, retrograde expulsions and pseudoarthroses[63]. As a result of these complications, surgeons have advocated the augmentation of PLIF with internal fixation[18]. One questions the potential benefits of these systems, as they themselves carry a high complication rate which outweighs their benefits[19,66]. The earlier users of PLIF had little in the way of instrumentation augmentation, yet managed to produced exceptionally good results.

Its role in the case of spinal stenosis[30], or post-chemonucleolysis[55], needs to be reconsidered. The long-term results of decompression for spinal stenosis are favourable[27]. Post-chemonucleolysis back pain in the majority resolves rapidly[61], and the early intervention with PLIF may be unnecessary. The author has found in the final analysis of the PLIF that it is a difficult technical procedure, time consuming with long a learning curve and fluctuating fortunes. It is noteworthy that, in what is effectively a tribute to the PLIF, many workers have developed interbody fusion cages going for the 'disc substitution'.

At the time of going to press the author has performed two pilot studies involving 51 cases of interbody fusion cages. Technically the Ray threaded fusion cage involves more operative surgical manoeuvres and bulkier instrumentation. The cage does not always follow the proposed trajectory line of the disc with occasional mal-placement. Two cases of L5 nerve root injury have resulted from distraction. The Titanium shell has a smaller surface area for bone integration, although one case in which a re-operation was necessary did reveal some bone formation through the cage. Five cases have undergone MRI scanning and all have produced artefact and failure of confirmation of bony fusion. Imaging sequences need re-analysis[36]. Gadolinium images have revealed a marked reduction of post-operative intra-spinal enhancement, supporting the theory of stability with less adhesion formation.

The Stryker Ogival Cages are easier to insert, aligning themselves ideally within the intra-discal space and relying on precision fit. The use of hydroxylapatite coating should add to the osseous bonding and the greater surface area will facilitate the fusion. No complications have occurred in the Ogival group.

In both studies there have been no mechanical failures, retrograde expulsion, aseptic or septic loosening of cage or graft. Both systems have provided immediate short term stabilisation without the need of additional instrumentation, a faster operating time, lower morbidity and shorter in-patient stay.

Evaluation of the clinical outcome is continuing. The early results are encouraging, with an impression of superior outcomes compared to more conventional fusion techniques and the likelihood of reduced pseudoarthrosis rate for both single and multiple level fusions. As with all new operations, salvage procedures are mandatory and in the case of interbody fusion cage failure, the author proposes reverting back to the posterior lumbar interbody fusion.

6. References

1.   F.H. Albee, *J.A.M.A.* **57** (1991) 885.
2.   Bak, Interbody Fusion System, Smith & Nephew Surgical Limited, Cambridge, CB5 8PB.
3.   W.J. Betts, J. Bone Joint Surg. **47-B** (1965) 593.
4.   H.G. Blume, *Clin. Orthop.* **193** (1985) 75.
5.   N. Bogduk, W. Tynan, A.S. Wilson, *J. Anat.* **132** (1981) 39.
6.   J.W. Brantigan, P.C. McAfee, B.W. Cunningham, H. Wang, C.M. Orbegoso, *Spine* **19** (1994) 1436.
7.   J.W. Brantigan, A.D. Steffee, *Spine* **18** (1993) 2106.
8.   A. Brieg, Adverse Mechanical Tension in the Central Nervous System. An analysis of cause and effect. Relief by Functional Neurosurgery, (Almqvist & Wiksell International, Stockholm, 1978)
9.   W.P. Bunnell, *J. Paediat. Orthop.* **2** (1982) 469.
10.   R.B. Cloward, *J. Neurosurgery* **10** (1953) 154.
11.   R.B. Cloward, *Clin. Orthop.* **154** (1981) 74.
12.   E. Colhoun, *J. Bone Joint Surg.* **70-B** (1988) 267.
13.   J.S. Collis, *Clin. Orthop.* **193** (1985) 64.
14.   S.D. Cook,, J.E, Dalton, E.H. Tan, W.V. Tejeird, M.J. Young, T.S.Whitecloud III, *Spine* **19** (1994) 1856.
15.   H.V. Crock, *Clin. Orthop.* **165** (1981) 157.
16.   A.F. DePalma, R.H. Rothman, *Clin. Orthop.* **59** (1968) 113.
17.   R.A. Deyo, Proceedings of the Degenerative Lumbar Spine. Lund, Sweden 1992.
18.   P. Enker, A.D. Steffee, *Clin. Orthop.* **300** (1994) 90.
19.   S.I. Esses, B.L. Sachs, V. Dreyzin, *Spine* **18** (1993) 2231.

20. J.H. Evans, *Clin. Orthop.* **193** (1985) 38.
21. G.E. Friedlaender, *J. Bone Joint Surg.* **69-A** (1987) 786.
22. A. Fugimaki, H.V. Crock, G.M. Bedbrook, *Clin. Orthop.* **165** (1982) 164.
23. K. Gill, S.L. Blumenthal, *Acta Orthop. Scand. Suppl.* **251** (1993) 108.
24. K. Gill, J.P. O'Brien, *Spine* **18** (1993) 1885.
25. A.E. Goodship, S.A. Wilcox, J.S.Shah, *Clin. Orthop.* **196** (1983) 61.
26. G.J. Groen, *Am. J. Anat.* **188** (1990) 282.
27. A. Herno, O. Airaksinen, T. Saari, *Spine* **18** (1993) 1471.
28. R.H. Hibbs, *N.Y. State J. Med.* **93** 1013.
29. R.H. Hibbs, *JAMA* **69** (1917) 787.
30. C.G. Hutter, *Clin. Orthop.* **193** (1985) 103.
31. I.A. Jaslow, *Surg. Gynaec. Obstet.* **82** (1946) 215.
32. P. Kambin, *Mt. Sinai J. Med.* **58** (1991) 159.
33. M.E. Katz, S.L. Teitelbaum, L.A. Gilula, *et al. Invest. Radiol.* **23** (1988) 447.
34. S. Kuslich, *Orthop. Clin. North Am.* **22** (1991) 181.
35. F. Lange, *Am. J. Orthop. Surg.* **8** (1910) 344.
36. H. Leclet, *Eur. Spine J.* **3** (1994) 240.
37. C.K. Lee, N.A. Langrana, *Spine* **9** (1984)574.
38. P.M. Lin, R.A Cautilli, M.F.Joyce, *Clin. Orthop.* **180** (1983) 154.
39. G. Lundborg, B. Rydevik, *J. Bone Joint Surg.* **55-B** (1973) 390.
40. G.W.C. Ma, *Clin. Orthop.* **193** (1985) 57.
41. W. Mercer, *Edinburgh Med. J.* **9** (1936) 545.
42. A.L. Nachemson, *Neurosurg. Clin. N. Amer.* **2** (1991) 785.
43. A.L. Nachemson, *Spine* **14** (1989) 555.
44. A. Naylor, *Ann. R. Coll. Surg.* **31** (1962) 91.
45. P.H. Newman, *J. Bone Joint Surg.* **37-B** (1955) 164.
46. H.E. Pedersen, C.F.J. Blunck, E. Gardner, *J. Bone Joint Surg.* **38-A** (1956) 377.
47. R.C. Quinnell, H.R. Stockdale, *Spine* **6** (1981) 263.
48. C.D. Ray, in *The Artifical Disc*, ed. M. Brock, M. Mayer, K. Weigel (1991).
49. C.D. Ray, Le Clerq, Proceedings International Intradiscal Therapy Society, Aberdeen (1994).
50. S.D. Rolander, *Acta Orthop. Scand. Suppl.* **90** (1966)
51. P.G. Roofe, *Arch. Neurol. Psychiat.* **44** (1940) 100.
52. R.H. Rothman, F.A. Simeone, *The Spine*, 2nd Ed. (W.B.Saunders Co., Philadelphia, 1982)
53. S. Sacks, *Clin. Orthop.* **44** (1966) 163.
54. N.A. Schechter, M.P France, C.K. Lee, *Orthopaedics* **14** (1991) 447.
55. R. Sepulveda, A.P. Kant, *Clin. Orthop.* **193** (1985) 68.
56. E.H. Simmons, S.K. Bhalla, *J. Bone Joint Surg.* **51-B** (1969) 225.
57. J.W. Simmons, *Clin. Orthop.* **193** (1985) 85.
58. R.N. Stauffer, M.B. Coventry, *J. Bone Joint Surg.* **54-A** (1972) 756.

59.   T. Toyone, K. Takahashi, H. Kitahara, M. Yamagata, M. Murakami, H. Moriya, *J. Bone Joint Surg.* **76-B** (1994) 757.

60.   J.A. Turner, M. Ersek, L. Herron, Haselkorn, D Kent, M. Ciol, A. Deyor, *JAMA* **268** (1992) 907.

61.   D. Wardlaw, in *Lumbar Spine Disorders*, Vol. 1, ed. R.M. Aspden, R.W. Porter, (World Scientific, Singapore, 1995) 167.

62.   J. Weinstein, B.Rydvik, *Seminar Spinal Surgery* **2** (1989) 100.

63.   T.F. Wetzel, H. La Rocca, *Spine* **16** (1991) 839.

64.   A.A. White, C. Hirsch, *Acta Orthop. Scan*d. **42** (1971) 482.

65.   B.R. Wiltberger, *Clin. Orthop.* **35** (1964) 69.

66.   K. Yashiro, T. Homma, Y. Hokari, Y. Katsumi, H. Okumura, A.Hirano, *Spine* **16** (1991) 1329.

CHAPTER 14

CLINICAL TRIAL TO INVESTIGATE STABILISATION OF THE SPINE

J.C.T. Fairbank, H. Frost and J. Wilson-Macdonald

1. Introduction

This chapter is a resumé of a protocol which we have presented to the Medical Research Council of the United Kingdom for a multicentre trial to investigate the value of spinal fusion and spinal stabilisation for chronic low back pain. It has not yet been accepted by the MRC. This protocol represents over two years work by the authors, and we are grateful for the input provided by many spine surgeons and physiotherapists in the UK and abroad, as well as those in this city and elsewhere with expertise in the establishment of large multi-centre trials. Clinical trials are only able to answer a limited set of questions. This protocol is designed to satisfy the (very reasonable) demands of public health doctors and health purchasers for evidence that this type of intervention is effective in the management of chronic back pain. It is not designed to demonstrate that one surgical technique is better than another. These questions can only be tackled if this trial demonstrates a clear advantage of surgical treatment over non-surgical rehabilitation.

2. Purpose

The aim of the Spine Stabilisation Trial is to establish whether or not surgical treatment of patients with chronic back pain by spinal stabilisation (fusion or ligamentous stabilisation) is more or less effective than less costly non-operative intensive rehabilitation treatment in achieving a worthwhile relief of symptoms. We propose a prospective, randomised, controlled trial of patients being considered for spinal fusion. The trial will be primarily based in the UK. We plan to recruit up to 1000 patients with follow-up for at least 2 years and will take five years to recruit sufficient patients, to follow them up, and to analyse the results. Stratification will allow for 3 diagnostic groups, and account for recognised confounding factors. Outcome will be measured by a variety of disability and satisfaction questionnaires, as well as functional capacity. There will be an economic evaluation. The surgical arm will permit a wide variety of stabilisation techniques to be evaluated and the non-operative arm will involve a standard functional restoration programme which will be similar in the different centres. The trial is the pragmatic testing of currently available management strategies in as broad clinical confines as possible based on the uncertainty principle. It incorporates a range of outcome measures to ensure the applicability of the results in the clinical and wider health service context.

3. Background

The management of patients with chronic low back pain has always been controversial. Investigation of surgical treatment of back pain has been recognised as a major national priority by the NSIS Standing Group on Health Technology. There is little consensus over the aetiology of back pain, and a wide variety of classification systems have been proposed. The economic costs of back pain, both to the individual patient, their families, employers and health service purchasers are well known, particularly as back pain tends to affect individuals who are otherwise fit and of working age. It is generally agreed that a large proportion of patients can be managed with conservative measures, the efficacy of some methods having support through controlled trials of variable quality[44]. When conservative treatment fails, spinal fusion is offered to some patients. The rationale for surgery, reported results and complications are variable, so that there is substantial uncertainty regarding the effectiveness of surgical treatment and the selection of patients for operation. The importance of developing evidence-based medical techniques has been emphasised by the Cochrane Collaboration (of which we are participants), and Orthopaedics and Physiotherapy are recognised as an important part of this process.

Spinal fusion was originally developed for the treatment of tubercle, and was later extended into the management of spinal deformity due to poliomyelitis, and idiopathic and congenital scoliosis. It has been used for the management of back pain from the earliest days. The treatment has been criticised for many years, and its results subject to numerous reviews, the most recent being that of Turner *et al.*[46]. Even this detailed analysis has been contested by other groups reviewing the same papers[9,49]. There are wide variations in practice in different medical cultures, although a recent study has shown an almost direct relationship between the numbers of spinal operations performed each year and the number of orthopaedic and neurosurgeons per head[3]. A wide variety of spinal fusion techniques are used, and there is no well recognised method of identifying which is the most appropriate for each patient[39]. Health service purchasers require evidence for the effectiveness and cost-effectiveness of alternative health care procedures to promote rational decision making. The scientific basis for spinal fusion has been strongly questioned, and recently various authors have advocated that a controlled trial of spinal fusion should be performed[6,15,46]. The time is now ripe to establish whether or not spinal fusion has any advantage over the very active conservative treatment of chronic low back pain advocated by Mayer and others[35]. Mayer compared a functional restoration regime versus non-intervention on a group of patients including those with previous failed back surgery as well as those thought unsuitable for surgery. Unfortunately the study was not randomised, but included a control group of patients who could not be funded for the programme. No satisfactory trial of conservative therapy has been carried out on patients with chronic back pain suitable for surgical treatment.

There are considerable methodological problems in conducting trials of surgical techniques, although this is being achieved for carotid endarterectomy, with valuable clinical results[4,17] and in the field of back pain, a non-randomised trial of the surgical treatment of herniated disc has been completed, with a 10 year follow-up of patients, whose results are widely quoted[48]. For example, it is difficult or impossible to keep the patient or metrologist 'blind' from the nature of the intervention. It may be difficult to persuade a patient that surgery and non-operative treatment are reasonable alternatives and the surgeon may come under pressure from patients in the conservative group to offer surgery. Surgeons vary widely in their selection of patients, and it is difficult to standardise surgical techniques, particularly in a multi-centre study. Pollock has discussed some of the problems associated with controlled trials of surgical procedures[42], including the importance of establishing rules for stopping a trial.

In the preparatory discussions for this trial it became clear that where some surgeons used spinal fusion, others used the Graf technique (see below for explanation of this method). A three-way trial of rehabilitation *vs.* fusion *vs.* Graf stabilisation was considered, but the Graf users, pleased with their results, felt unable to offer spinal fusion as a true surgical alternative to their patients. Similarly those surgeons still using spinal fusion were unhappy with a technique unsupported by refereed publications. If a trial was established using either one of these techniques, the other surgeons and their patients would be lost to the trial. The solution is to offer a trial of spinal stabilisation *vs.* rehabilitation in which the surgeon will indicate before randomisation whether Graf stabilisation (or equivalent) or spinal fusion will be offered to the patient (if allocated surgery). This will allow an overall comparison of all those allocated surgery versus all those allocated rehabilitation, and unbiased subgroup comparisons of each type of surgery versus randomly allocated rehabilitation subgroups.

4. Reported results of spinal fusion

These have been reviewed recently by Turner *et al.* who found a wide variation in both the clinical success rate(16-95 %) and the rate of pseudarthrosis(56-100 %)[46]. This review was not able to identify any obvious advantage in using instrumentation, and suggested that these techniques may increase the level of complications. A recent review of the Steffee fixation system (a modern pedicle screw system) by its originator claims an 80 % clinical success rate and 92 % fusion rate[45]. This paper suffers most of the methodological defects identified by Turner *et al.*, including a significant dropout rate and the use of invalidated outcome measures. A paper in the same edition of the journal 'Spine' points to the difficulties in identifying pseudarthrosis on plain radiographs compared with operative exploration[2]. Overall agreement in this study was 69%, with a 42% false positive rate, and 29% false negative rate in a group of patients with a 90% fusion rate found at operation. For this reason, in this study, we have decided to confine our outcome measures to validated patient satisfaction measures, although 'obvious' pseudarthrosis rates will be recorded. The Turner review has been criticised in turn by Dorey *et al.* who, by defining subgroups of patients and calculating confidence intervals have arrived at different conclusions[9].

5. Graf stabilisation

Graf, of Lyon, has developed an alternative method of stabilising the spine without using a fusion. This involves the insertion of pedicle screws into each vertebra to be stabilised. These are then attached to one another with Dacron loops. This method has the theoretical advantages of both simplicity (to surgeons familiar with the insertion of pedicle screws) and avoiding the problems of the bone graft donor site. Further, it does not prevent a spinal fusion being attempted at a later date. This device is now available for use in several countries, but has not been subjected to a controlled trial. Graf has a personal series extending over 4 years which has yet to be published in a refereed journal. In the UK, a personal series of 50 patients treated by Mr Alan Gardner has been reviewed by an independent assessor, Grevitt. These patients were reviewed at 19-36 months and the results await publication. 72% of patients are reported as 'excellent or good'. The mean Oswestry Disability Index fell from 59% preoperatively to 31% at review, which is comparable with the reported series on spinal fusion (personal communications).

6. Non-operative management

In the past, rest has been advised for the conservative management of back pain, but recent research has demonstrated that there is no real advantage in resting for more than three days after an acute attack of low back pain[8]. Active exercise programmes to reduce the disabling effects of low back pain[8] are now advocated[24,47]. Many other treatments are available for the management of back pain but there are very few prospective controlled trials that have satisfied scientific scrutiny. Koes *et al.* reviewed over 50 prospective studies in an attempt to assess the effectiveness of exercise and manipulative therapy for patients with back pain and concluded that the quality of the papers they reviewed was poor[26,28]. They then carried out a well controlled study comparing manipulative therapy, traditional physiotherapy, GP management and placebo physiotherapy treatment for patients with at least a six weeks history of non-specific back and neck pain. At the 12 month follow up assessment they found that beneficial results were gained in both the physiotherapy and manipulative therapy group but further trials were necessary to determine long term effects in patients with more specific conditions[27]. Unfortunately, patients included in this study were not comparable with those suitable for spinal stabilisation surgery. There is now a considerable amount of evidence to suggest that the physical effects of back pain can be complicated by non-physical factors such as stress and anxiety. Due to the disability and psychological distress caused by chronic back pain multidisciplinary intensive rehabilitation programmes have been developed. Most of the intensive programmes include back schools, exercise, muscle training, relaxation, psychological techniques and some form of traditional physiotherapy *i.e.* heat, manual therapy or electrotherapy. The majority of papers demonstrate beneficial results[5,20,23,29,30,33,34,36,37] with a minority reporting negative effects of treatment[1] or poor results at long term follow up[19]. However, the evidence is inconclusive due to the variation in patient population and diagnosis, duration and severity of symptoms and treatment intervention.

A psychological approach to the treatment of chronic pain has been described by Fordyce[13]. Research has shown this approach to be effective for the management of chronic back pain[11,31,32,40]. A meta-analysis by Flor *et al.* included 65 studies that evaluated the efficacy of multidisciplinary treatments for chronic back pain[12]. They concluded that pain management programmes including psychological intervention are superior to no treatment, traditional therapy and medical treatment and that the benefits were stable over time. Unfortunately, few centres in the UK offer pain management programmes and those that do are reserved for the most chronically disabled patients who have failed to improve with any other type of intervention, including spinal surgery. Studies aiming to assess the efficacy of physical and psychological treatment have not overtly included patients that would be considered suitable for spinal stabilisation surgery. It is, therefore, unclear whether this group of patients, primarily complaining of chronic back pain and disability, would benefit from conservative intervention. Most patients presenting for stabilisation surgery have usually undergone various forms of traditional therapy and are therefore unlikely to respond to further traditional treatment. The most convincing evidence for the treatment of patients with chronic LBP supports the use of multidisciplinary pain management programmes.

7. Proposed conservative treatment strategy

A protocol based on paced activity, education and psychological intervention is planned. We recognise that there could be variations in the programmes offered by different centres (as is the case in surgical methods), but since few centres have an established programme, we expect that the recommended programme (Figure 1) will be complied with by the participants. This consists of a three week intensive programme with patients attending daily from Monday to Friday. A follow-up session should be arranged at 3 months and 6 months. Local patients would attend on a daily outpatient basis and those from further away would be accommodated in nearby guest houses to reduce costs. Training in the recommended programme will be provided to physiotherapists and psychologists from the participating centres. The aims of the programme would be to reduce functional disability and increase every day activity. Education sessions would include the following: The consequence of inactivity; Depression and anxiety; The consequence of persistent pain and repeated treatment; The importance of pacing activity, reward for activity and appropriate rest; Short term and long term goals setting; Rationalisation of medication; Pain/Illness behaviour. Physical treatment would include individualised progressive exercise programmes based on the patients baseline capability. All exercise sessions would be paced to avoid over activity and hydrotherapy would be included if available in the centre carrying out the treatment. This programme would require medical supervision, a minimum of 1 full time physiotherapist, a part time clinical psychologist and clerical support.

8. Plan of investigation

8.1. Eligibility

All patients with more than 12 months history of chronic back and referred pain are eligible for the trial. This includes patients who have had previous root decompression or discectomies, but not those who have had previous attempts at surgical stabilisation of the spine. As far as possible the patients for admission to the trial should have been fully investigated by the techniques normally used by the responsible surgeon. These criteria are designed to be inclusive rather than exclusive, and to reflect the reality of everyday clinical decisions in this area.

8.2. Uncertainty Principle

Patients will be eligible when both the clinician and patient are uncertain as to whether surgical stabilisation or rehabilitation is indicated. Thus if the clinician or patient is absolutely certain of the successful outcome of stabilisation in a particular patient, then that patient should not be entered into the trial. On the other hand if the clinician or patient is convinced that spinal stabilisation will be unsuccessful, then again the patient is ineligible for the trial.

8.3. Diagnostic groups

Although it has proved difficult to achieve consensus on diagnostic groups, it is clear that most reported series of patients treated with lumbar fusion fall into a restricted area of supposed pathology, and there are three groups which can be recognised by the participating clinicians with little or no confusion. Diagnostic grouping is recognised as a major confounding factor in all treatments used in back pain patients. The clinical sub-groups we plan to use are listed below. Most surgeons expect the best results in group (b) and the worst in group (c) and in general this view is supported by the many open ended studies that have been published. This classification represents a pragmatic approach to the diversity of clinical problems seen in this group of patients.

(a) **'discogenic' back pain.** Patients with one or more degenerate lumbar discs identified as being symptomatic by whatever means normally employed by the responsible clinician, not falling into one of the other groups.

(b) **Spondylolysis and spondylolisthesis** of one or more levels of the lumbar spine, including degenerative spondylolisthesis. The type of spondylolisthesis will be recorded (lytic, isthmic, degenerative).

(c) **'post-laminectomy syndrome'.** Where a patient has had previous surgery to decompress lumbar nerve roots, usually by discectomy. Patients previously treated with chemonucleolysis or percutaneous discectomy will be included in this group. Patients who have had previous lumbar spinal fusions will be ineligible for the trial.

8.4. Randomisation

The patients will be randomly allocated to one of two treatment strategies: (1) A conservative treatment strategy; (2) A spinal stabilisation strategy. Trial participants will be provided with a proforma, which will record the principal data required prior to randomisation. The surgeon responsible will follow a standard protocol to introduce the patient to the trial. The patient will be seen and assessed by the trial physiotherapist, who will use a written as well as a verbal explanation, with a video, which can be taken home by the patient, to help in gaining consent. Randomisation will be performed at a preadmission, with a further assessment. This is because it is likely that there will be some delay between the surgeon deciding that surgical stabilisation is appropriate and the date of admission (because of waiting lists). This will allow an assessment of the stability of the

WEEK 1	Monday	Tuesday	Wednesday	Thursday	Friday
9.00- 9.30	Welcome and Introduction	Set baseline exercise programme	Stretching	Stretching	Stretching
9.30-10.00	To include aims of programme and orientation	As above	Function of the spine. Causes of pain. Mechanism of acute and chronic pain	Healing and effects of disuse on the body systems	Goal setting. Potential difficulties and relevance to daily activities
10.00-10.45	Assessment and Questionnaires	As above	Circuit	Circuit	Circuit
10.45-11.15	Coffee	Coffee	Coffee	Coffee	Coffee
11.15-12.00	Measurements	Introduction to goal setting	Posture: Positioning in walking, standing, sitting and sleeping	Drugs and medication	Overview of problems related to pain
12.00-1.00	Hydrotherapy	Hydrotherapy	Hydrotherapy	Hydrotherapy	Hydrotherapy
1.00-2.15	LUNCH and Rest	LUNCH and Rest	LUNCH and rest	LUNCH and rest	LUNCH and rest
2.15-3.00	Importance of paced exercise. Explain over activity and under activity cycle.	Circuit	Ergonomic workshops including specific problems	Stretching and relaxation	Stretching and relaxation
3.00-3.15	Tea	Tea	Tea	Tea	Tea
3.15-4.00	Video assessment	Stretching and Relaxation	Stretching and Relaxation	Principles of hydrotherapy	Discussion of week end plan and goals
4.00-4.30	Discussion	Discussion	Discussion	Discussion	
Evening reading	Read information sheets	Goal setting. Think about short term and long term goals	Think about activity that you would like to do in free time next week	Read information sheets and week end plan	

Figure 1. Outline of recommended rehabilitation programme, week 1 (continued overleaf).

WEEK 2	Monday	Tuesday	Wednesday	Thursday	Friday
9.00-9.30	Stretching	Stretching	Stretching	Stretching	Stretching
9.30-10.00	Welcome back and week end report	Posture and gait	Treatments for pain. Understanding medical treatment and therapy.	The role of your friends relatives and partners	The effect of anxiety, stress, irritability and anger (CS)
10.00-10.45	Circuit	Circuit	Circuit	Circuit	Circuit
10.45-11.15	Coffee	Coffee	Coffee	Coffee	Coffee
11.15-12.00	The importance of being fit.	Posture and gait	Video. Back fire	Understanding joints	Making changes in your life. Invite partner or friend
12.00-1.00	Hydrotherapy	Hydrotherapy	Hydrotherapy	Hydrotherapy	Hydrotherapy
1.00-2.15	LUNCH and Rest	LUNCH and Rest	LUNCH and rest	LUNCH and rest	LUNCH and rest
2.15-3.00	Explanation of investigations and X rays.	Circuit	Understanding illness behaviour	Stretching and relaxation	Stretching and relaxation
3.00-3.15	Tea	Tea	Tea	Tea	TEA
3.15-4.00	Stretching and Relaxation	Stretching and Relaxation	Stretching and Relaxation	Free time for planned activity	Discussion of week end plan and goals
4.00-4.30	Discussion	Discussion	Discussion	Discussion	
Evening reading	Goal setting. Think about short term and long term goals	Read information sheets. Plan activity for free time	Read information sheets	Read information sheets and consider week end plan	Consider what you have learnt so far. Try to concentrate on changing body posture and focus on what you can do

Figure 1. Outline of recommended rehabilitation programme, week 2 (continued overleaf).

WEEK 3	Monday	Tuesday	Wednesday	Thursday	Friday
9.00-9.30	Stretching	Stretching	Stretching	Stretching	Stretching
9.30-10.00	Welcome back and week end report	Plan for increased pain in future	Free activity	Video assessment	Plan for setbacks and maintenance(CS)
10.00-10.45	Circuit	Circuit	As above	Circuit	Circuit
10.45-11.15	Coffee	Coffee	Coffee	Coffee	Coffee
11.15-12.00	Adjusting or resetting goals. Setting long term goals	Lifting and handling techniques	Stretching and relaxation	Considering body posture. Review videos.	Time for individual discussion with CS and final assessment
12.00-1.00	Hydrotherapy	Hydrotherapy	Hydrotherapy	Hydrotherapy	Final discussion
1.00-2.15	LUNCH and Rest	LUNCH and Rest	LUNCH and rest	LUNCH and rest	
2.15-3.00	Circuit	Circuit	Learning to cope with pain. Reinforcement	Stretching and relaxation	
3.00-3.15	Tea	Tea	Tea	Tea	
3.15-4.00	Stretching and Relaxation	Stretching and Relaxation	Circuit	Plan goals to be achieved by follow up appointment	
4.00-4.30	Discussion	Discussion	Discussion	Discussion	
Evening reading	Goal setting. Reassess goals short term and long term	Read information sheets. Plan activity for free time	Write a plan of problems you may have now or in the future and how you are going to tackle them on your own	Read information sheets and consider week end plan	Consider what you have learnt so far. Try to concentrate on maintaining and achieving your goals.

Figure 1. Outline of recommended rehabilitation programme, week 3. (contd.)

principal outcome measures before intervention. Treatment should follow randomisation as soon as possible. Randomisation will be by the Oxford Clinical Trial Service Unit, who can be contacted by telephone (working hours only in UK) or fax 24 hours a day. Randomisation will be carried out using a specially written programme, which will ensure balance between the treatment groups with respect to various prognostic factors: 1) Participating Centre; 2) Age; 3) Gender; 4) Occupation/spouse's occupation (social class); 5) Work status; 6) Smoking; 7) Litigation; 8) Oswestry Disability Score; 9) Psychological scores (Zung; MSP); 10) Duration of symptoms; 11) Clinical classification (one only) (degenerative disc disease; spondylolisthesis (lytic, isthmic, degenerative); post-laminectomy syndrome); 12) If allocated to 'stabilisation', type of surgery planned (Fusion; Graf (or similar) stabilisation). The randomisation form is shown in Figure 2, and the randomisation protocol summarised in Figure 3.

---

1) Participating Centre   _____
2) Hospital number   _____
3) NHS number (if available)   _____
4) Family Name   _____
5) Given name   _____
6) Date of birth   day___ month___ year_____
7) Sex   Male/female
8) Occupation/spouse's occupation   _____
9) Work status   H'wife/working/not working/unemployed
10) Current regular smoker   Yes/no (or unsure)
11) Litigation(involved with solicitors or equivalent)   Yes/no (or unsure)
12) Oswestry Disability Score   _____%
13) Psychological scores -   Zung   _____
14)   -   MSP   _____
15) Duration of symptoms   _____months
16) Clinical classification (one only)   degenerative disc disease
                                                       spondylolisthesis(specify type)
                                                          (lytic, isthmic, degenerative)
                                                          post-laminectomy syndrome

17) If allocated to 'stabilisation', treatment planned
                                                       Fusion
Levels to be fused: L1/2; L2/3; L3/4; L4/5; L5/S1; Other

                                                       Graf (or similar) stabilisation
Levels to be stabilised: L1/2; L2/3; L3/4; L4/5; L5/S1; Other

Figure 2. Randomisation form

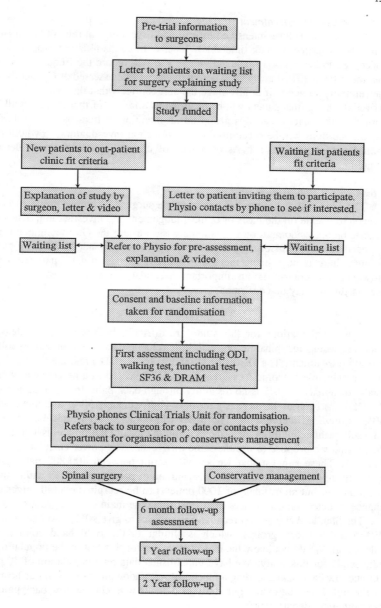

Figure 3. Randomisation protocol

8.5. A conservative treatment strategy

This would include intensive physical and psychological rehabilitation (see appendix 1 for the proposed 3 week timetable). Ideally, this rehabilitation programme should be under the supervision of a single individual who will record the frequency and duration of treatment for the final analysis. These patients will be assessed at 6 monthly intervals by the referring surgeon. If at any stage the surgeon feels that the case for offering surgery is overwhelming, that patient will be recorded as a failure of therapy, but will be analysed with the other patients in this group on an intention to treat basis. The basis for these clinical decisions will be scrutinised by the principal investigators, to whom this decision should be justified on a basis of a lack of clinical improvement or deterioration in symptoms.

8.6. A spinal stabilisation strategy

The type and technique and extent of the surgical technique are left to the referring surgeon to decide on the basis of clinical judgement and investigation. The surgeon must indicate before randomisation if he or she wishes to use the Graf technique (or similar) as opposed to spinal fusion. No formal attempt is to be made to identify pseudarthrosis because there is no reliable method to identify pseudarthrosis apart from reoperation. However reoperation is an important secondary outcome measure, during which pseudarthrosis may be confirmed.

8.7. Power

Power calculations for this study are difficult, because of the wide variations of published results for spinal fusion, with little reliable data on the outcomes following non-operative treatment. The Oswestry Disability Index (ODI) and the Shuttle Walking Test are the principle outcome measures. The ODI is scored as a percentage, where 100% is totally disabled, and 0% is no disability through back pain. In spinal fusion series where the ODI has been used, there is a mean of approximately 50%, and most report a fall to 30% following intervention. The MRC Chiropractor Trial took 4% on the ODI as a clinically meaningful difference (incidentally the mean ODI on admission to this trial was 24%), and we propose to use the same difference. The power calculations are set out in Table 1. These suggest that we should recruit between 400-800 patients to detect a clinically relevant difference. The distribution of patients recruited within the subgroups is unknown, but an estimate of 1000 patients to be recruited overall, gives a reasonable chance of detecting differences in at least some the main clinical groups.

The Shuttle Walking Test requires 850 subjects to give 90% power to show a 50 metre difference between groups, which is similar to the right hand column of the ODI calculation. We do not know the expected values for this test in the population of patients admissible for this study. We have unpublished data on a population of 30 patients with chronic low back pain attending a functional restoration programme in our hospital, as well as the published data from our study of patients with chronic low back pain attending a physiotherapy department[45].

Table 1: Power calculations for Oswestry Disability Index (to detect a change in ODI from 50%-30% compared with 50%-34%) showing the approximate numbers of patients required.

	Standard Deviation = 10	Standard Deviation = 15
P<0.01		
90% Power	350	800
80% Power	300	600
P<0.05		
90% Power	300	600
80% Power	200	450

8.8. Recruitment

Initially the trial will be conducted by UK surgeons, but it is likely that surgeons in the rest of Europe, as well as Australasia, and Canada, and possibly elsewhere may become involved. How successful we shall be in recruiting patients to this study remains to be seen, and this factor alone is the main reason for conducting a pilot study. We believe that we have facilitated procedures from the point of view of the surgeon, and the physiotherapist/metrologist will have a key role to play in encouraging recruitment. The experimental use of the video is to try to harmonise the process of explanation in different centres, to standardise recruitment, and to explain and to reassure patients as to the validity and nature of the study, the process of informed consent and the uncertainty principle. The pilot study will determine whether or not the trial continues, and whether we have to look abroad to achieve sufficient patients into the study. We recognise that all trials ultimately depend on the enthusiasm of their participants. All the participants are aware of this important fact. The video consent is an important part of promoting patient confidence (because we have taken the trouble to make it, and (we hope) because of the quality of explanation on the video). We are concerned that without the video there may be a wide variation in the admission process, and that patients may be lost from the trial unnecessarily.

We have encouraged participants to approach patients on their waiting lists to 'sound them out' as to whether they would be prepared to join the trial when they are called up for preoperative assessment. We are unsure how successful this strategy will prove, but we hope it will discourage a delay between starting the trial and recruiting the first patient (all surgeons have waiting lists). We have also encouraged the surgeons to discuss the trial with patients that they are seeing in their clinic at the moment who are being listed for spinal fusion.

8.9. Ethical Committee approval

This has been obtained in Oxford (COREC 94.204; approved: 10/8/94), and the participating Centres are currently presenting the trial to their Local Research Ethics Committees.

9. Health Economics

The substantial costs of back pain to individuals, the health service and society in general have been well documented[7,25]. However, there have been few attempts to calculate the costs or cost-effectiveness of specific interventions. Deyo *et al.*[7] and Powell *et al.*[43] have examined resource use associated with spinal fusion, but in both instances the studies were quite different from that in the present proposal. They were performed in the United States, compared fusion with other surgical interventions rather than non-surgical interventions, and looked at patient populations (elderly and paediatric respectively). In this proposal, the costs and cost-effectiveness of a conservative treatment strategy compared with a spinal stabilisation strategy will be examined as part of the trial. In each case the main focus of the analysis will be on within-trial differences in costs and cost-effectiveness. The proposed evaluation, therefore, addresses a number of important economic issues. First, it will provide actual data rather than estimates of the treatment paths, resource use and cost variations associated with surgical treatment of back pain (although the probability of receiving surgical treatment for back pain is comparatively low, surgical treatment accounts for a large proportion of the estimated costs of back pain). Second, it will provide information on cost-effectiveness of therapies in an area where data on effectiveness and on costs are currently inadequately researched.

9.1. Costs

Data will be collected on (a) the costs of the recommended 3-week programme (including staffing, training, equipment and accommodation) at each centre; (b) the costs of the surgical interventions, including hospital stay and subsequent outpatient visits; (c) the costs of subsequent interventions, such as reoperation or other related health care use. Costs associated with general practitioner consultations will be collected by means of retrospective postal questionnaires to trial participants. As there is likely to be substantial variations in costs between centres, the cost analysis will report all results using: (i) resource use and cost data from each centre, and (ii) resource use data from each centre and standard cost data based on average costs reported across all participating centres.

It is likely that patients and their families will bear some of the costs of chronic back pain. The retrospective postal questionnaire will also be used to collect data on the economic impact of chronic back pain of a patient's household, including equipment and adaptations, and the impact on informal carers. It is anticipated that health service and family cost data will be collected for each individual enrolled into the trial. 100 % sampling will increase the power of the cost-effectiveness analysis and enable a full statistical analysis of cost data in parallel with effectiveness data. Indirect costs associated with return to paid employment within one year of intervention (an outcome measure of the trial) will be evaluated, using baseline and one-year data on employment status in each trial arm. These indirect costs will be reported separately from direct costs.

9.2. Effectiveness

Cost-effectiveness will be defined in terms of the primary outcome measures of the trial (especially the ODI, SF36 and shuttle walking tests). Thus cost-effectiveness will be expressed as a net cost per unit change in disability score and per metre gain in walking distance. These cost-effectiveness ratios will be calculated for each arm of the trial, in order to assess the *incremental* cost per unit ODI or metre shuttle walking test.

10. Outcomes

10.1. Steering Committee
The trial will be directed by the applicants and others.

10.2. Data Monitoring Committee
This is a vital part of the trial. This group, who will not be involved in submitting patients to the trial, will monitor the results of treatment in each group. If a clear advantage or disadvantage to a particular group appears during the trial in the view of the Data Monitoring Committee, then they will advise the Steering Committee, who can then decide whether to stop or modify the trial accordingly. The statistical bounds for stopping the trial will be established before the trial starts. Analysis will be on an intention to treat basis. As far as possible analysis will be extended into sub-groups of patients and surgical techniques, but it is unlikely that an answer to the question of what is the optimum fusion technique will be obtained.

10.3. Follow-up
A minimum 2 year follow-up is planned. It is appreciated that longer term follow-up is ideal, and if possible this will continue after initial reporting.

10.4. Outcome measures and size of difference to be measurable
These measures will be made at pre-specified points by a Physiotherapist at each centre not involved in the treatment of the patient. The measurements will be made at initial assessment, at randomisation (if more than 3 months from initial assessment), 6 and 12 months post treatment, and then annually.

10.5. Oswestry Disability Index
This scale has been in widespread use for fifteen years both in assessment and as an outcome measure and will form one of the principal outcome measures for this study. It has been well validated[1,10].

10.6. Shuttle walking test
This was developed at Loughborough for the assessment of respiratory function. It has subsequently been used and validated as an outcome measure for patients with chronic low back pain. This test requires the patient to walk up and down a ten metre course identified at each end by two cones inset 0.5 metre from each end to avoid the need for abrupt changes in direction. The explanation to the patient is standardised and played from a tape at the start of the test. Accuracy of the timed signal is assured by the inclusion on the tape recording of a calibration period of one minute. The speed at which the patient walks is dictated by an audio signal played on the tape recorder. In the first minute the patient is

required to walk up and down the walkway three times (amounting to a distance of 30 metres). The following minute requires the patient to walk faster and complete 40 metres within the time dictated by the audio signal from the tape recorder. The speed and distance is then increased each minute until the end of the test. To assist the patient in establishing the routine of the test, the assessor walks alongside the patient for the first minute. No form of encouragement is permitted during the test. The patient has to reach the end of the walkway before a tone sounds. Initially even the slowest walker can achieve this, but gradually as the interval between the tones decreases the subject is forced to speed up. The observer counts the number of times the subject passes between the cones. Eventually the subject cannot reach the other cone before the tone sounds. Even if the end point may be controversial on one pass, it rapidly becomes obvious in the next pass or two that it has been achieved. The endpoint of the test is either: 1) by the patient stopping because of increased pain or fatigue, or 2) by the operator, if the patient fails to complete a shuttle in the time allocated. This test has been shown to be sensitive to change in patients with chronic low back pain[14]. This test will provide the main 'objective' test of function for patients in this study. A 50 metre improvement (5 passes) will be considered the minimal difference between the treatment arms that is of clinical significance (this represents an improvement in speed and endurance).

10.7. Other 'Objective' tests

A battery of simple standardised physical tests have been developed and tested for reliability in patients with chronic pain[18,50]. Clear standardised instructions should be given by each assessor to enhance reliability. Of these tests, the following two tests would be included in this trial: 1) Stand up sit down: 2 minutes. 2) Stair climbing: 2 minutes.

10.8. SF36

This general health questionnaire has been validated recently in two British studies[16,21]. Patients with back pain have worse quality of life scores than patients with any of the other common medical complaints measured in this study[22]. Recent quality of life measures have been reviewed by this group, and the SF36 seems to offer the best generic health status instrument for this trial[22].

10.9. Work status

This is a notoriously difficult outcome measure to use, but in terms of justifying the costs and value of intervention in this age group is important. A positive outcome is return to paid employment within 1 year of intervention.

11. Secondary outcome measures

11.1. Implant failure

This will be recorded in all cases where an implant fails within a two year follow up.

11.2. Pseudarthrosis

This is widely perceived as an important outcome measure. However there are considerable difficulties in reliably establishing failure of fusion[2]. It is also recognised that clinical failure is not always related to failure of fusion. It will be recorded if there is clear evidence of pseudarthrosis, and this is reported by the physician responsible. A systematic review of radiographs is not planned, as this trial is designed to test current clinical practice.

11.3. Neurological damage

Clear clinical or neurophysiological evidence of post-treatment neurological damage.

11.4. Reoperation rate

This is an unequivocal outcome measure. However there is scope for considerable variation between centres, and it has therefore been included as a secondary outcome measure.

12. References

1. D. Baker, P. Pynsent, and J. Fairbank, *The Oswestry Disability Index revisited,* in *Back pain: New Approaches to Rehabilitation and Education,* M. Roland and J. Jenner, Editor. (Manchester University Press, Manchester, 1989) p. 174.
2. S. Blumenthal and K. Gill, *Spine* **18** (1993) 1186.
3. D. Cherkin, *et al., Spine* **19** (1994) 1201.
4. Clinical Alert, *National Institute of Neurological Diseases and Stroke publication.* (1991).
5. R. Cutler, *et al., Spine* **19** (1994) 643.
6. R. Deyo, *Spine* **18** (1993) 2153.
7. R. Deyo, *et al., Spine* **18** (1993) 1463.
8. R. A. Deyo, A. K. Diehl, and M. Rosenthal, *N. Eng. J. Med.* **315** (1986) 1064.
9. F. Dorey, P. Grigoris, and H. Amstutz, *J. Bone Joint Surg.* **76-B** (1994) 1.
10. J. Fairbank, *et al., Physiotherapy* **66** (1980) 271.
11. H. Flor and N. Birbaumer, *Comprehensive assessment and treatment of chronic back pain patients without physical disabilities.* (Proceedings of the VIth World Congress on Pain: 1991)
12. H. Flor, T. Fydrich, and D.C. Turk, *Pain* **49** (1992) 221.
13. W.E. Fordyce, in *Behavioural Methods for Chronic Pain and Illness.* (C.V. Mosby Co., Illinois, 1976).
14. H. Frost, *et al., Brit. Med. J.* **310** (1995) 151.
15. J. Frymoyer, *Spine* **18** (1993) 2147.
16. A. Garratt, *et al., Brit. Med. J.* **306** (1993) 1440.
17. E.C.S.T.C. Group, *Lancet* **337** (1991) 1235.
18. V.R. Harding, A.C.d.C. Williams, and P.H. Richardson, *Pain* (1994).

19.   J. Harkapaa, *et al.*, *Scand. J. Rehab. Med.* **21** (1989) 81.
20.   R. Hazard, *et al.*, *Spine* **14** (1989) 157.
21.   C. Jenkinson, A. Coulter, and L. Wright, *Brit. Med. J.* **306** (1993) 1437.
22.   C. Jenkinson, L. Wright, and A. Coulter, in *Quality of life measurement in health care: a review of measures and population norms for the UK SF-36*. (Health Services Research Unit, Department of Public Health and Primary Care, University of Oxford, Oxford, 1993).
23.   K. Kellet, D. Kellet, and L. Nordholm, *Physical Therapy* **71** (1991) 283.
24.   W. Kermond, R.J. Gatchel, and T. Mayer, in *Contemporary Conservative Care for Spinal Disorders,* eds. T.G. Mayer, V. Mooney, and R.J. Gatchel, (Lea & Febiger, Philadelphia, London, 1991).
25.   J. Klaber Moffett, *et al.*, in *Back Pain: Its Management and Cost to Society*. (Centre for Health Economics, York, YO1 5DD, UK, 1995).
26.   B. Koes, *et al.*, *Brit. Med. J.* **303** (1991) 1298.
27.   B. Koes, *et al.*, *Brit. Med. J.* **304** (1992) 601.
28.   B. W. Koes, *et al.*, *Brit. Med. J.* **302** (1991) 1572.
29.   S. Kohles, *et al.*, *Spine* **15** (1990) 1321.
30.   I. Lindstrom, *et al.*, *Physical Therapy* **72** (1992) 279.
31.   S. J. Linton, *Pain* **21** (1985) 289.
32.   S. J. Linton, *Behavioural Research Therapy* **25** (1987) 313.
33.   C. Manniche, *et al.*, *Pain* **47** (1991) 53.
34.   T. Mayer, R. Gatchel, and N. Kishino, *Spine* **10** (1985) 482.
35.   T. Mayer, *et al.*, *JAMA* **258** (1987) 1763.
36.   H.J. McQuade, J.A. Turner, and D.M. Buchner, *Clin. Orthop.* **233** (1988) 198.
37.   R. Mitchell and G. Carmen, *Spine* **19** (1994) 633.
38.   R. Mulholland, *J. Bone Joint Surg.* **76-B** (1994) 517.
39.   A. Nachemson, *Acta Orthop. Scand.* **64 Suppl 251** (1993) 130.
40.   M.K. Nicholas, P.H. Wilson, and J. Goyen, *Pain* **48** (1992) 339.
41.   G. Oland and G. Tveiten, *Spine* **16** (1991) 457.
42.   A. Pollock, *Brit. J. Surg.* **80** (1993) 964.
43.   E. Powell, *et al.*, *Spine* **19** (1994) 1256.
44.   W. Spitzer, *Brit. J. Indust. Med.* **50** (1993) 385.
45.   A. Steffee and J. Brantigan, *Spine* **18** (1993) 1160.
46.   J. Turner, *et al.*, *JAMA* **268** (1992) 907.
47.   G. Waddell, *Spine* **12** (1987) 632.
48.   H. Weber, *Spine* **8** (1983) 131.
49.   A. White, *et al.*, *Spine* **19** (1994) 109.
50.   A.C.d.C. Williams, *et al.*, In *Patient vs outpatient pain management: Results of a randomised controlled trial. Proceedings of the 7th World Congress on pain.* (1993).

CHAPTER 15

MANAGEMENT OF SPINAL STENOSIS

J.E. Nixon

1. Introduction

Lumbar spinal stenosis is a clinical condition which arises when one or a number of nerve roots in the spinal canal are compressed because of narrowing of the spinal canal. Such narrowing may be caused in a variety of different ways ranging from disc protrusion to neoplastic infiltration and Paget's disease but traditionally the term lumbar spinal stenosis is reserved for degenerative narrowing of the spinal canal. Narrowing of the spinal canal is a normal ageing process, particularly at the L4/5 and L5/S1 levels as marginal osteophytes grow on the facet joints and margins of the vertebral body adjacent to the disc. In the vast majority of individuals, however, this is of no consequence since at skeletal maturity (when degenerative change begins) they have developed a large spinal canal with sufficient reserve capacity to accommodate future narrowing. In those individuals who start off with a smaller spinal canal or in whom the degenerative change becomes more advanced for one reason or another, the likelihood exists that they will eventually suffer pressure on one or more nerve roots in the cauda equina.

The onset is usually insidious in the fifties and sixties but may be more rapid in the forty and fifty year old when degenerative change is combined with sudden failure of the intervertebral disc. There may be a long history of back pain but symptoms of sciatica are intermittent initially and brought on, for instance, by exercise or posture. In the later stages of spinal stenosis the sciatic pain may be constant and eventually the whole cauda equina may be involved at one or more levels resulting in bladder and possible bowel disturbance.

The factors responsible for degenerative spinal stenosis are illustrated briefly in Figure 1. The difference between the symptoms and signs of spinal stenosis compared with those of prolapsed intervertebral disc and peripheral vascular disease are summarised in Tables 1 and 2.

In this chapter, I shall describe briefly the methods of conservative treatment used in a group of 149 patients and the results achieved. I shall then describe the surgical treatment of a separate group of 72 patients with spinal stenosis in whom the results of surgery were assessed immediately post-operatively and subsequently at periods extending up to 10 years. The immediate post-operative result will be compared with the long term results. Finally, I shall review briefly a small series of 12 patients who were referred because of failure of the first operation and who underwent further surgery. The results will be presented and finally recommendations made for the assessment and management of patients who have failed to respond to spinal decompression together with an analysis of the reasons for failure in this small series. The total number of patients reported here

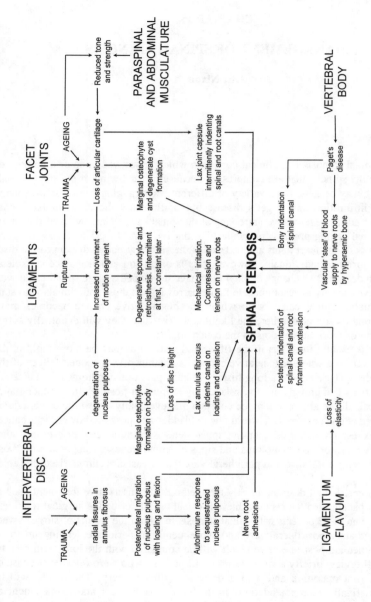

Figure 1. Factors responsible for degenerative spinal stenosis.

Table 1. Differential diagnosis of symptoms.

		Spinal Stenosis	Prolapsed Intervertebral Disc	Peripheral Vascular Disease
Onset		Insidious	Rapid	Slow
Age		Over 50	30 - 50	Over 60
Precipitating factor		Fall or lifting	Lifting or bending	Smoking - previous MI or CVA
Leg pain	character	Neurogenic - numbness aching tingling pins & needles	Neurogenic - sharp shooting 'electric shock' pins & needles	Cramping Dull ache
	location	Sciatic distribution often including foot	Sciatic distribution often including foot	Calf or buttock
	induced by	Standing - postural: severe Walking - ischaemic: mild	Standing, walking, sitting: severe Bending, lifting: mild	Walking or other exercise
	relieved by	Sitting or squatting Lying in foetal position	Lying flat on boards	Rest, (standing, sitting or lying down)
	'march'	Up or down	Usually down	Absent
	sitting	Relieves leg pain	Aggravates leg pain	No difference
	cycling	Relieves leg pain	Aggravates leg pain	Aggravates leg pain
	lateralisation	Unilateral or bilateral	Usually unilateral	Unilateral or bilateral
Back pain		Usually present	Present or absent	Present or absent (non-contributory) Present in feet in severe ischaemia
Night pain		Present in 20%	Absent	
Weakness		May appear with exercise or present at rest when severe	May be present at rest	Rare but muscle may go into spasm
Bladder and/or bowel disturbance		Present when severe	Present when central disc prolapse	Absent

Table 2. Differential diagnosis of signs.

	Spinal Stenosis	Prolapsed Intervertebral Disc	Peripheral Vascular Disease
Posture	Simian stance.	Loss of lordosis with sciatic scoliosis when acute.	Normal.
Sitting	Comfortable.	Painful, tends to sit on one buttock.	Comfortable.
Lying	Unable to lie prone.	Comfortable if still.	Comfortable.
Walking	Leans forwards, maybe supported by walking sticks.	Antalgic gait favouring pain-free side.	Walks normally as far as claudication distance.
Spinal mobility	Normal flexion. Reduced extension. Reduced lateral flexion in lateral stenosis.	Reduced flexion. Normal extension. Reduced lateral flexion away from side of scoliosis.	Normal.
Neurological examination: sensory	Deficit appears or increases with exercise or present at rest when severe.	Deficit present at rest, dermatomal distribution.	Usually none. Peripheral neuropathy (stocking distribution) of diabetes sometimes present.
motor	Deficit appears or increases with exercise or present at rest when severe.	Myotomal distribution at rest.	Rare. Muscle may cramp and tighten on exercise.
reflexes	Absent or diminished ankle reflex is most consistent finding.	May be diminished or lost ankle reflex.	Normal.
Lasègue's sign	Negative.	Positive, crossed when severe	Negative.
Vascular examination: peripheral pulses	Normal.	Normal.	Absent or diminished. May disappear with exercise.
bruits	None.	None.	Present - aortic, femoral or popliteal.
General features	Neuropathic ulcers on feet. May have coexistent vascular disease in this age group.	No ulcers. No vascular disease.	Trophic ulcers on feet; cardiac failure; arcus senilis; diabetes; previous cerebro-vascular incident.

therefore comprises 233 patients with spinal stenosis followed up over a 10 year period. The factors responsible for the production of spinal stenosis are illustrated in Figure 2.

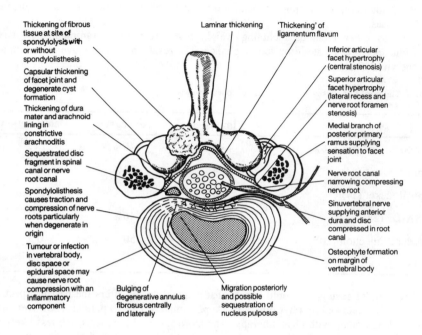

Figure 2. This diagram illustrates at least 14 possible causes of nerve root compression. It also shows the innervation of the facet joints, dura and annulus fibrosus through which pain impulses are mediated.

2. Conservative management

Of the 149 patients with spinal stenosis managed conservatively, 86 were male and 63 female. The average age of the males was 63 and the females 60 and this represents an older age group than the surgical group because of the number of elderly patients in the conservative group who were considered unfit for surgery. The results are based on a clinical assessment at the beginning and end of treatment. Although patients in the surgical group were usually treated conservatively in the first instance, they have been excluded from the series of conservative treatment for sake of clarity.

The methods of conservative treatment employed were as follows:-

a) Bed rest in hospital with or without traction for a period of two weeks. (This option is no longer available.)

b) Spinal corset for three months.
c) Plaster jacket or plastic jacket for six weeks.
d) Non-steroidal anti-inflammatory drugs for a period of three months.
e) Epidural injection.
f) Physiotherapy, consisting of heat, ultrasound and isometric back strengthening exercises.
g) Various other methods including weight loss, swimming, transcutaneous nerve stimulation and a Yates drop foot appliance. The results of conservative treatment are shown in Table 3.

Table 3. The results of conservative treatment of spinal stenosis

	Improved	No change	Deterioration
Enforced bed rest (26)	40%	46%	14%
Spinal corset (84)	74%	23%	3%
Spinal jacket (17)	65%	18%	17%
NSAIDs (28)	46%	46%	8%
Epidural injection (20)	50%	50%	0%
Physiotherapy (32)	66%	25%	9%

From these results, it would appear that a spinal corset offers the best prospect of improvement followed by physiotherapy. Approximately 1 in 10 patients, however, will notice a deterioration with physiotherapy. The more severe the stenosis, the less likely an epidural injection is to be effective. In the present climate of bed shortage, it seems unjustifiable to offer patients hospital bed rest with only a 40% prospect of improvement and a 14% prospect of deterioration. Although some patients reported improvement after regular swimming and other patients reported an improvement with weight loss the numbers were too small to reach any conclusions. The ankle-foot orthosis used to control a drop-foot deformity in a small group of patients unsuitable for surgery improved their gait but did not reduce their pain.

3. Surgical management

72 patients with spinal stenosis were managed by surgical decompression. There were 47 males and 25 females, of which 72% of the males and 85% of the females had degenerative stenosis. The commonest type of stenosis in the males was a combined disc degenerative stenosis and the commonest type in the females was a degenerative spondylolisthesis, usually at the L4/5 level.

3.1. Surgical technique

A small number of patients in the early part of the series underwent decompressive laminectomies, but the majority were treated by segmental spinal decompression using a partial undercutting facetectomy. The involved level can be approached by using a 3 cm mid-line incision. Mobility of this skin permits the incision to be moved proximally and distally to allow a more extensive incision into the dorsolumbar fascia, preserving the interspinous ligament. The L4/5 and L5/S1 levels can be identified by visualising the sacrum. Higher levels were identified using X-ray control.

Figure 3(a) illustrates the lower part of the lamina with the medial part of the inferior facet, the shaded area is the area to be removed. Figure 3(b) shows the appearance

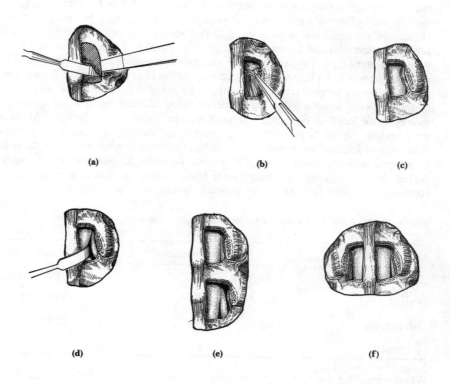

Figure 3. Surgical procedure for a decompressive laminectomy.

following the removal of this bone. The ligamentum flavum was reflected and excised. Figure 3(c) shows the prominent medial aspect of the superior facet of the vertebra below which is compressing the nerve root in the lateral recess. This was excised using an osteotome to reveal the nerve root as illustrated in Figure 3(d). When required, this operation can be performed at two levels on one side (Figure 3(e)) or, alternatively, bilaterally at the same motion segment (Figure 3(f)). Note that the important interspinous and supraspinous ligaments are preserved and utilised for the reattachment of the dorso-lumbar fascia. The intervertebral disc is preserved whenever possible. Post-operatively the patient can be mobilised on day one and allowed home if comfortable and mobile. A post-operative corset is provided for a few weeks to help control any post-operative discomfort.

3.2. Results of surgical decompression on sciatic pain

The objective assessment of the results is complex. Improvement noted on electrophysiological testing and post-operative imaging using CT or MRI scanning to assess the adequacy of decompression may be gratifying for the surgeon, but the patient's own verdict on the operation is what counts. This series therefore relies on the patient's subjective assessment of the results of surgery combined with a post-operative review of the pre-operative clinical signs. The initial post-operative assessment took place within one month of surgery and a long term re-assessment was made at an average of 3 years and 10 months following surgery (range 13 months to 10 years). 83% noted either improvement or total relief of sciatica following segmental spinal decompression whilst a very slight increase in the incidence of sciatica was noted in a small proportion of patients. At the long term review, further improvement was noted in the majority of patients with residual symptoms of sciatica, sometimes up to two years after decompression. The total number of patients enjoying complete relief of sciatica therefore doubled during the follow up period. 39% of patients experienced some minor symptoms, usually a minor and brief recurrence of sciatic pain following strenuous physical activity (Table 4).

Table 4. Results of surgery on sciatic pain at initial and final assessment.

	Initial assessment	Long-term assessment
Total relief	22%	44%
Partial relief	61%	39%
No change	15%	12%
Increased	2%	5%

When comparing the initial with the final post-operative result, 39% of patients noted further improvement with the passage of time whilst 19% experienced some increase in sciatic pain, though not sufficient for them to consider further surgery. A stable result was found in the remaining 42%

3.3. Results of surgical decompression on low back pain

The majority of patients continued to experience some low back pain despite decompression. It is important to emphasise to the patients pre-operatively that the operation is not performed to relieve back pain but to relieve sciatic pain. Overall, at the initial assessment 69% of patients noted improvement or resolution of back pain and this was maintained in the long term in the vast majority of patients (Table 5). Just over 20% of patients noted some further improvement between the initial and final assessments, though 26% reported a gradual deterioration and 53% were unchanged.

Table 5. Effects of surgery on low back pain at initial and final assessment.

	Initial assessment	Final assessment
Resolved	13%	25%
Reduced	56%	37%
No change	26%	32%
Increased	5%	5%

3.4. Changes in neurological signs following spinal decompression

Almost 70% of patients noted improved strength in the legs following spinal decompression and 60% of patients noted improved sensation in the legs (Table 6). It is important to note that 14% of patients thought the legs were weaker following decompression and in 18% of patients the sensory deficit increased post-operatively. Clearly patients need to be advised of this possibility prior to surgery. The majority of patients with sensory or motor deterioration following surgery were nonetheless pleased with the results of spinal decompression since they were relieved of sciatic pain.

Table 6. Changes in neurological function following spinal decompression

	Motor power	Sensation	Reflexes
Return to 'normal'	11%	38%	30%
Improved	58%	19%	2%
No change	7%	14%	10%
Deterioration	14%	18%	14%
Normal pre-operatively	10%	11%	44%

4. Prognostic indicators

By comparing the patients who fared well with those who fared less well following surgery, an attempt was made to identify those factors which would allow a surgeon to predict pre-operatively the outcome of surgery.

Unfortunately no correlation was found between the outcome and the following factors:

a)	age at presentation
b)	occupation
c)	type of stenosis
d)	delay in presentation
e)	operative findings
f)	levels decompressed
g)	Number of different levels decompressed.

Though no clear prognostic indicators were identified to predict the long term results, the impression was gained that patients with multiple level stenosis tended to deteriorate over the years. When stenosis involved one segment only, the results tended to remain stable during the long term follow up period.

5. Revision Surgery

A group of 12 patients, separate from those reported above, were referred because of failure of previous spinal decompression. Each of the patients underwent further surgery and their clinical data and the final results are given in Table 7. If no persistent nerve root compression was identified then no further surgery was recommended. The reasons for the failure of the initial operation(s) are

Inadequate decompression	75%
Failure to recognise developmental stenosis	17%
Inappropriate surgery (wrong level)	8%

In the vast majority of patients, the lateral recess or nerve root canal had not been adequately decompressed. The second most common cause of failure of the initial operation was only removing a slightly bulging disc instead of decompressing a developmentally narrow lateral recess. This was because narrowing of the lateral recess had not been recognised and the condition was thought to be due entirely to a disc prolapse. Generally these patients did well following appropriate surgery. This study confirmed what is already well known that following multiple spine operations, patients with psychosocial problems, including depression, or those with arachnoiditis or with litigation pending do less well following surgery. However, 7 out of the 12 patients who underwent further surgery were satisfied with the results and were pleased with the decision to re-operate.

The assessment of patients who have failed to respond to spinal decompression is

Table 7 Repeat surgery on 12 patients. The reasons, final operation, interval between operations and the final outcome

Case	Age at final op.	Initial operation	Reason for failure	Final operation	Interval	Total ops.	Final result, time from last op.
1	43	L4/5 laminectomy	Inadequate transverse decompression	Discectomy + lateral recess decompression	3 months	3	Dissatisfied 5 yrs
2	43	L4/5 laminectomy	Inadequate longitudinal decompression	L3/4 laminectomy + discectomy	1 year	2	Dissatisfied 4 yrs
3	57	L5/S1 discectomy	Inadequate transverse decompression	L5 laminectomy + lateral recess decompression	6 months	2	Satisfied 7 yrs
4	58	L3/4 & L4/5 discectomy	Inadequate transverse decompression	L4/5 laminectomy + lateral recess decompression	6 months	2	Satisfied 1 yr
5	54	L1/2 discectomy	Inappropriate surgery	L2/3 discectomy + partial laminectomy	3 months	2	Dissatisfied 5 yrs
6	48	L4/5 partial decompression	Repeatedly inadequate decompression	L4/5 laminectomy + lateral recess decompression	6 years	4	Dissatisfied
7	29	L4/5 discectomy	Unrecognised developmental stenosis	L4/5 laminectomy	3 years	2	Dissatisfied 7 yrs
8	39	L4/5 & L5/S1 exploration	Unrecognised developmental stenosis	L4/5 laminectomy	8 years	2	Satisfied 4 yrs
9	65	L4/5 discectomy	Inadequate transverse decompression	Emergency L4/5 laminectomy + lateral recess decompression	11 years	3	Satisfied 2 yrs
10	55	Right L4/5 discectomy	Inadequate transverse decompression	L4/5 laminectomy + left L4/5 discectomy	3 years	2	Satisfied 4 yrs
11	42	L4/5 discectomy & foramenotomy	Borderline inadequate decompression	L5 laminectomy + lateral recess decompression	9 years	2	Satisfied 3 yrs
12	59	L4/5 discectomy, L5/S1 exploration	Inadequate transverse decompression	L4/5 laminectomy + lateral recess decompression	12 years	2	Satisfied 2 yrs

complex. For those who find algorithms helpful, Figure 4 suggests a method of assessing patients in whom sciatica predominates following spinal decompression and Figure 5 an approach for patients in whom low back pain predominates.

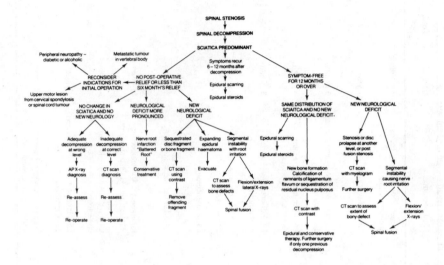

Figure 4. Algorithm to indicate which category of patient may be suitable for reoperation for those who fail to respond to spinal decompression because of persistent or recurrent sciatic pain.

Acknowledgement: I am most grateful to Edward Arnold, Division of Hodder and Stoughton, for permission to reproduce figures 1 - 4, figures 6-10 and 12-15 from Spinal Stenosis edited by John E. Nixon, 1991.

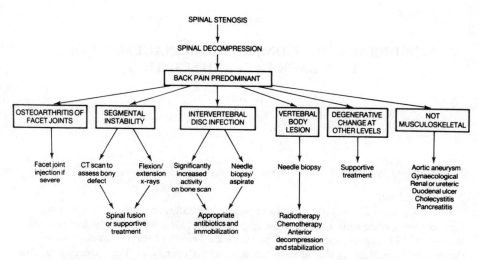

Figure 5. Algorithm to indicate which patients may be suitable for reoperation after failing to respond to spinal decompression because of persistent or recurrent back pain.

CHAPTER 16

EPIDURAL INJECTIONS IN THE MANAGEMENT OF LOW BACK PAIN AND SCIATICA

K. Bush

1. The history of epidural injections

1.1. 1900 - 1960

In 1901 Sicard[102] was the first to recognise the safety of the caudal route for the introduction of anaesthetic agents into the epidural space. One week after he had presented the results of his animal experiments to the Biological Society of Paris, Cathelin[23] described the use of a cocaine caudal anaesthetic in a hernia operation. The extension of this technique to the treatment of sciatica was popularised by Caussade and Queste[24] in 1909. In 1929 Gasser and Erlanger[42] demonstrated that dilute solutions of local anaesthetic agents could differentially block small unmyelinated nerve fibres without affecting larger motor and proprioceptive fibres.

The technique was introduced to Britain by Evans[37] in 1930. He reported encouraging results after the injection of 100 ml of both 1% procaine and normal saline. In 1944 Kelman[64], using equally large volumes, carried out 486 injections in 116 patients with sciatica. He particularly noted that the relief of pain outlasted the expected period of activity of the injected local anaesthetic.

Cyriax[29] popularised this technique, advocating it in the treatment of patients with lower lumbar intervertebral disc lesions with nerve root pressure, with or without neurological signs. He used 0.5% procaine hydrochloride in normal saline and contended that 50 ml was just as effective as 100 ml, supporting this claim with radiological and post-mortem evidence. Following the introduction of corticosteroids in the 1950s and the discovery of their strong anti-inflammatory potential, steroids were soon introduced into the epidural space. The finding of evidence of inflammation, both macroscopic and histologic, in relation to nerve roots compressed by prolapsed disc material[11,16,43,44,73,77,78,81,92,96] provided the necessary rationale.

1.2. 1960 - 1985

There are a great number of papers which deal with the use of epidural injections in the management of lower back pain and sciatica[4,6,15,17,18,25,30,47,48,49,57,59,60,62,69,82,98,99,101,112,116,119,121]. Unfortunately, most of these are reviews and so the conclusions are unreliable. In 1962 Barry and Hume-Kendall[4] drew attention to the lumbar route as a means of introducing corticosteroid into the epidural space in an attempt to reduce inflammation of nerve root sheaths.

2. Prospective, randomised, double blind, placebo-controlled studies

A literature review uncovers six such studies: Dilke *et al.*[33], Brevik *et al.*[13] and Ridley *et al.*[91] are in favour of epidural injections in the management of lower pain and sciatica while Snoek *et al.*[103], Cuckler *et al.*[28] and Klennerman *et al.*[67] are not.

2.1. Studies in favour of epidural injections

Dilke *et al.*[33] treated 100 consecutive in-patients thought to have lumbar nerve root compression.

The criteria for admission to the trial were the presence of pain in the distribution of the sciatic or femoral nerves accompanied by one or more of the following features:
1. Painful limitation of sciatic or femoral nerve stretches.
2. Sciatic scoliosis.
3. An appropriate neurological deficit.

Those in the treatment group received one or two epidural injections of 80 mg methylprednisolone in 10 ml of normal saline via the lumbar route as described by Barry and Hume-Kendall[4]. Those in the control group received superficial injection into the interspinous ligament of 1 ml of normal saline. Assessment during admission and at 3 months revealed statistically highly significant differences in respect of relief of pain and resumption of normal occupation in favour of the group treated by extradural injection.

Breivik *et al.*[13] treated a complex group of 35 patients with incapacitating chronic lower back pain and sciatica unresponsive to conservative treatment for several months to several years. Eleven patients had previously undergone surgery for prolapsed intervertebral discs, 32 patients had radiculography with metrisamide before the epidural injections showing arachnoiditis in 8, prolapsed intervertebral discs in 8, no abnormality in 11 and inconclusive findings in 5. The study construction was a cross-over, patients either receiving a caudal injection of 20 ml bupivicaine 0.25% with 80 mg prednisolone first or 20 ml bupivicaine 0.25% with 100 ml of normal saline first. If there was no improvement after the first injection, up to three injections of the alternative were given. The results were evaluated according to the effects on the severity of pain, anaesthesia, Lasegue's test, paresis, spinal reflexes and sphincter disorders. Nine (56%) of the 16 patients to receive the corticosteroid first had significant pain relief whereas 5 (26%) of the 19 patients who received saline first had significant pain relief. Eleven of the remaining patients subsequently had corticosteroid and 8 (73%) experienced significant pain relief. Thus, 63% of those who received corticosteroid and 26% of those who received saline experienced pain relief and objective neurological improvement sufficient to enable the patient to return to work or be rehabilitated to other work ($P=0.05$).

Ridley *et al.*[91] treated 30 patients on an outpatient basis. Patients were selected on the basis of a clinical history and signs consistent with sciatic nerve root compression defined as pain in a sciatic distribution with numbness or paraesthesia in the area or an appropriate neurological deficit. Patients with low back or leg pain and restriction of straight leg raise alone were not admitted. This was again a crossover study, patients either receiving an epidural injection of normal saline with 80 mg methylprednisolone via the lumbar route as described by Barry and Hume-Kendall[4] or 2 ml of normal saline into the interspinous ligament. After one week the same injection was repeated if there was little or no benefit. If lack of improvement persisted for another week and placebo had been injected initially, patients were given active treatment. Patients were independently assessed for rest and walking pain on the visual analogue scale and straight leg raise at 1, 2 and 4 weeks. Significant differences in pain relief were seen between the two groups at 2 weeks. This benefit disappeared for 6 (35%) patients within six months of treatment although 11 (65%) successfully treated subjects had sustained improvement up to this time. It was concluded that out-patient epidural injections of corticosteroid are a useful short-term means of pain relief in sciatica but probably have little long-term effect on the natural history of symptoms. Two patients suffered the complication of dural tap.

2.2. Studies not in favour of epidural injections

Snoek *et al.*[103] studied 51 patients suffering from sciatica of 2 to 36 weeks duration. All patients had signs, symptoms and myelographic abnormalities consistent with lumbar disc herniation and in particular, all patients had a neurological deficit. Each patient received an epidural injection, via the lumbar route, of 2 ml (80 mg) methylprednisolone or 2 ml normal saline. Patients were clinically assessed by the same neurologist before and between 1 to 3 days after the injection. This failed to demonstrate any statistical difference between the two groups and thus it was concluded that a single epidural injection of 80 mg of methylprednisolone was no more effective than a placebo in relieving chronic symptoms due to myelographically confirmed lumbar disc herniations.

Cuckler *et al.*[30] studied 73 patients with sciatica due to intervertebral disc herniation or spinal stenosis, confirmed radiologically (by myelography, CT scan or venography). Patients received 2 ml (80 mg) methylprednisolone acetate combined with 5 ml of 1% procaine or 2 ml normal saline combined with 5 ml 1% procaine, via the L3/4 lumbar route. Patients were reassessed within 24 hours for improvement of pain. This demonstrated no statistical difference between the groups. Those patients who had not responded to either injection within 24 hours received a second injection of methylprednisolone. Long-term follow-up averaging 20 months failed to demonstrate the efficacy of the second injection.

Although both of these studies discourage the use of epidural corticosteroids, their additional admission criteria indicated that all patients had both a neurological deficit and a significant myelographic defect. Such patients could be considered to be suffering from severe sciatica, and to be less responsive to conservative management. Secondly, assessments, including determination of spinal mobility and neurological deficit, took place between 1 and 3 days of the procedure. Such parameters are slow to improve and it is likely that changes may not be evident for several months. Pain, the most relevant parameter, may take up to 10 days to respond. Thirdly, only 2 ml and 7 ml volumes of methylprednisolone injection were administered on single occasions. It is questionable whether such volumes would always reach the appropriate nerve root on a single administration[20,115].

Klennerman[67] studied 74 patients suffering from unilateral sciatica of less than 6 months duration with or without neurological signs. They were treated in one of four ways receiving one lumbar epidural injection of:

1. 20 ml normal saline
2. 80 mg methylprednisolone in normal saline made up to 20 ml
3. 20 ml 0.25% bupivicaine solution made up with normal saline
4. Needling with a standard Touhy injection needle into the interspinous ligament but no injection.

The patients were re-assessed 2 weeks and 2 months after the procedure using a 100 mm visual analogue scale to quantify pain as well as the words mild, moderate or severe. Examination for lumbar flexion, using Schober's method, and straight leg raise was made. No statistical difference between the 4 groups could be demonstrated although, over-all, 75% of the in-patients improved or were cured. It was therefore concluded that the epidural injections achieved effects partially as a placebo and partially by virtue of the natural history of acute sciatica. Possibly a larger series would have reached statistical significance.

3. Therapeutic agents

3.1. Normal saline

Davidson and Robin[31] reported on 28 patients with sciatica who received large volumes (average 72 ml) of normal saline epidurally. They believed that nerve root pain was caused by the nerve root being compressed by hypertrophic tissue which was adherent to it. They ascribed their successful results to the mechanical disruption of adhesions and/or stretching of the nerve roots. Bhatia and Parikh[10] agreed with this analysis and claimed success in treating 108 patients with epidural injections of between 80-100 ml normal saline administered via the lumbar route. They also pointed out that normal saline was safer to use than local anaesthetic. Gupta *et al.*[51] also supported the use of normal saline after using, on average, 50 ml in a series of 23 patients suffering from sciatica.

There is thus the suggestion in the literature that epidural normal saline may influence the pathological processes by some mechanical means but no controlled studies have been carried out. Normal saline is certainly safe but is more commonly used as a carrying agent for local anaesthetic or steroids.

3.2. Local anaesthetics

Epidural local anaesthetics predominated in the management of lower back pain and sciatica before the introduction of steroids[24,26,29,42,64,102]. Cyriax[29] popularised the use of dilute solutions of local anaesthetic (0.5% procaine hydrochloride) first shown by Gusser and Erlanger[42] to block small unmyelinated nerve fibres differentially. Procaine hydrochloride was one of the first readily available local anaesthetics but of course there are many others today such as lignocaine hydrochloride, bupivicaine and so on. All of these can be used in low enough concentrations to avoid significant anaesthesia or paralysis of the lower limbs. As with procaine, the appropriate concentration of lignocaine is 0.5% but for bupivicaine it is 0.125%. If these concentrations are used it is possible for the patient to ambulate sooner rather than later, thus allowing the procedure to be performed on an out-patient basis. Having said this, bupivicaine has a very long half life and is particularly cardiotoxic. Thus inadvertent intrathecal or even intravenous administration would certainly result in a more profoundly disastrous situation than when using a shorter acting local anaesthetic. Cyriax[29] claimed to have carried out over 30,000 caudal epidural injections, using 0.5% procaine hydrochloride, and experiencing very few significant complications.

The means whereby local anaesthetic has apparently achieved relief of pain for periods greatly in excess of its normal duration has been a source of debate. It may be that whilst anaesthetized, and when able to move more freely again, the patient achieves a degree of self- manipulation. The other possibility is in the breaking of a pain cycle as suggested by Wall and Melzack[111].

3.3. Corticosteroids

Various steroid preparations first became available in the 1950s. Burn and Langdon[21] were able to demonstrate the depression of plasma cortisol levels for up to two weeks following the epidural administration of 80 mg and 160 mg of methylprednisolone.

Because of their strong anti-inflammatory effect there is extensive evidence to support the use of epidural steroids in the management of sciatica[11,15,43,44,66,73,77,78,81,86,92,96]. Most authors have described the use of methylprednisolone[6,13,28,33,48,67,101,103,112]. Despite these publications and the relatively common use of epidural steroids over the past 30 years, no pharmaceutical company actually has a licence which allows them to advocate the use of steroid preparations in the epidural space.

4. Variations of epidural anatomy, volume and the spread of injected fluids

Trotter[109], reporting a large post-mortem study, has described the inconsistency of the size and shape of the sacrum and particularly of the sacral hiatus. She also noted a variation in the lower limit of the dural sac from S1 to S3 and a range of canal volumes from 12 ml to 65 ml.

Evans[37] studied the cerebrospinal fluid pressure variations during injection and he recorded a rise up to 30 cm of water after 30 ml had been injected into the epidural space. Thus the epidural space is in fact a potential space and the introduction of fluid initially causes a rise in pressure, which is directly proportional to the volume of fluid introduced, until the fluid gradually disperses. MacIntosh and Bryce-Smith[76] have drawn attention to the variable connection between the epidural space and the paravertebral space via the intervertebral foramina. Further valuable information has been gained by contrast epidurography using urographin and sodium diatrizoate[72]. Emery and Hamilton[35] safely used epidurography on an out-patient basis.

An important investigation into the spread of solutions in the epidural space was carried out by Burn *et al.*[20] Using epidurography both via the lumbar and caudal routes, they concluded that the distribution of solutions in the epidural space was particularly related to the volume used and the site of injection, while the height and age of the patient, rate of injection and posture exerted no influence. Nonetheless, they did note wide variations in spread with a given volume via the same route. It was therefore impossible to predict the degree of spread accurately. However, clinical improvement following epidural injection for lumbosciatic syndromes did not appear to be correlated with a wide dissemination of the solution used and large volumes seem to confer no advantage. In particular, when using the lumbar route, the solutions tended to spread cephalad and rarely descended below L5, thus presumably not reaching pathology at the L5/S1 level. Further, the caudal administration of 20 ml of solution spread to L1 in general (Figure 1).

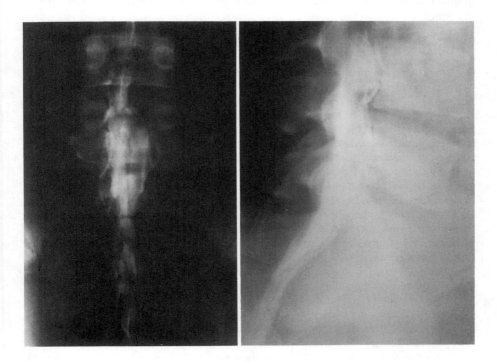

(a)   (b)

Figure 1. A caudal epidurogram demonstrating the spread of fluid in the epidural space. (a) an anterior-posterior view following the introduction of 8 ml Iohexol 300. (b) A lateral view taken 2 minutes after (a) demonstrating further spread of the contrast medium from the L4 to the L3 level.

5. The caudal versus the lumbar route

It has been argued that infection is more likely to be introduced via the caudal route being in close proximity to the perineum. However, this should not present a problem provided an appropriate aseptic protocol is adhered to. The caudal route offers a relatively extensive space for needle placement and thus a much reduced risk of dural tap over the lumbar route. This makes the caudal route safer as an out-patient procedure. However, the variation in sacral anatomy can result in failure and, for instance, extrasacral injection, in inexperienced hands. Caudally administered drugs will always reach the usual pathological levels of L5/S1, L4/5 and L3/4 provided an adequate volume of fluid is introduced whereas it has been shown that fluids introduced via the lumbar route tend to spread in a cephalad direction[20] and thus pathology situated caudad of the injection site may be missed. Alternatively, Barry and Hume-Kendall[4] have argued that the lumbar route allows for more precise placement, thus enabling the use of smaller volumes and higher concentrations of the drugs.

6. The safety and side-effects of epidural injections

It is noteworthy that the extensive literature previously reviewed does not report any serious complications[4,6,13,15,17,18,25,28,30,33,47,48,49,57,59,60,62,67,68,69,82,91,98,99,101,103,112,116,119,121]. In reviewing the reports on over 10,000 epidural injections prior to 1982, Corrigan *et al.*[27] point out that reports of major complications were excessively rare. Benzon[8] who also extensively reviewed the literature in 1986, concludes that epidural steroid injection is a safe procedure. Nonetheless the potential side-effects of epidural injections are quite serious, for instance if infection is introduced. There is an epidural venous plexus and intravenous injection of local anaesthetic in any volume can rarely lead to cardiovascular collapse. Bupivacaine with its long half life is particularly neuro- and cardiotoxic and it is now accepted that intrathecal administration of methylprednisolone preparations may lead to arachnoiditis[84], though only after a considerable number of repeated injections. However, if adequate precautions are taken and a meticulous technique adhered to, as should be the case with every invasive procedure, then the literature supports epidural injection as a safe procedure. In reviewing 1000 patients who had received lumbar epidural injections, mostly for lumbar disc derangement, Burn[19] reported that there were no complications apart from dural tap in less than 1% and occasionally mild hypotension.

There are also a multitude of minor side-effects which have been observed and reported. Headache can of course follow dural puncture but Abram and Cherwenka[1] have reported transient headaches immediately following epidural steroid injection in 8 out of 604 patients. Knight and Burnell[68] have reported Cushingoid facies in 2 patients and an acneform skin rash in 2 patients. However, these patients had received doses in the region of 350 mg of methylprednisolone acetate over a 3 day period which is far greater than that advocated by most authors. I have noted the occasional disruption of the menstrual cycle, transient increase in lumbosacral symptoms and transient facial flushing. The latter has been reported as a not infrequent side-effect of intra-articular steroid injection. Transient bladder dysfunction usually accompanies the use of higher concentrations of anaesthetic than is necessary to block the nociceptors[42] (*i.e.* more than 0.5% of procaine hydrochloride). Finally, prior to the injection of any drug, a history of allergy should always be enquired after and in particular that to dental anaesthetic injections.

7. A controlled study of caudal epidural injections of triamcinolone plus procaine in the management of intractable sciatica

While most authors are in favour of this technique, few have carried out well-designed, prospective, double blind trials to evaluate the procedure critically, and opinions remain conflicting[13,28,33,67,91,103].Conservative treatment consists of bed rest, analgesics, physiotherapy and epidural injections. In Bell and Rothman's[7] extensive review, however, the use of epidural injections was rejected on the basis of a single study. A well constructed study was therefore needed to ascertain the impact of caudal epidural injections on the quality of life in patients with sciatica.

7.1. Patients and methods

The inclusion criteria were based on the well recognised symptoms and signs indicative of lumbosacral nerve root compromise summarised by Cyriax[29] amongst others. These were root pain, exemplified by unilateral sciatica extending below the knee and associated with paraesthesia and root tension signs in the form of a positive straight leg raise. Patients were considered for the study with or without signs of root compression, *i.e.* neurological signs. The trial was of double blind, parallel group construction with neither patient nor assessor being aware of the injection content. The study procedure involved 2 caudal injections; the first following admission to the trial and the second after 2 weeks. The active therapy was a caudal injection of 25 ml containing 80 mg of triamcinolone acetonide in normal saline with 0.5% procaine hydrochloride. The placebo group received a caudal injection of 25 ml normal saline.

Subjective and objective assessments of the patients were made at each visit over one year. Subjective assessment comprised a specific symptomatology questionnaire designed by Grogono and Woodgate[50] to determine any effects upon the patient's lifestyle together with a visual analogue scale (VAS) and pain scale to define the degree of back and leg pain. Objective analysis was made by recording the angle of straight leg raise (SLR) measured using a Loebl goniometer[71].

7.2. Results

23 patients were entered. The average duration of symptoms prior to admission to the study was 4.7 months (range 1 - 13), with no significant difference between the active treatment and placebo group. 12 Patients received active treatment and 11 placebo.

5 Patients were withdrawn, 4 from the placebo group and 1 from the active group, due to deterioration of symptoms. This difference was not significant (chi-squared, $P = 0.4$). Of the 5 patients, 2 from the placebo and 1 from the active group underwent decompressive surgery, whilst the remaining 2 placebo patients were successfully managed with additional triamcinolone plus procaine epidural injections. At the 4 week visit the placebo treated group showed no significant changes in either objective or subjective measures. The actively treated group, however, demonstrated significant improvement in all aspects. Pain was significantly reduced ($P=0.02$) on both the VAS and pain scale, while lifestyles significantly improved ($P=0.02$). Physical improvement measured by the change in straight leg raise was significant ($P=0.01$). Between group analysis particularly showed a significant difference in SLR ($P=0.01$) and pain score ($P=0.06$). Between group analysis also showed a significant difference in SLR and pain score before and after the second injection and at 4 weeks: (for SLR $P=0.01$, for pain $P=0.01$, 0.06 and 0.06).

In broad terms, subsequent assessments demonstrated a statistically significant resolution of symptoms and signs in the placebo treated group, while the earlier benefit in the actively treated group was maintained or improved. Thus between groups analysis no longer showed significant difference for pain relief, although objective assessment of straight leg raising still showed a more significant benefit in the actively treated group ($P=0.01$) at 12 weeks.

7.3. Discussion

Sciatica, due to lumbosacral nerve root compromise, is a debilitating condition frequently afflicting otherwise healthy individuals. Pain and reduced mobility severely compromise their quality of life and are particularly disruptive to the working individual, when time off work may have unfortunate consequences. The aim of any therapy should be achievement of a normal lifestyle as soon as possible, whether it be by treatment of the underlying cause or merely symptomatic relief.

It is recommended that surgery should be used only when conservative management fails. However, there are no definite recommendations for when hospitalisation and surgical intervention should be considered[63]. Conservative management of this condition using caudal injections can, however, be conducted on an outpatient basis. Caudal injections are often beneficial; however, their role in the management of sciatica remains uncertain as discussed by Bell and Rothman[7].

Dilke *et al.*[33] supported the administration of epidural steroids via the lumbar route as an in-patient procedure. More recently, Ridley *et al.*[91] demonstrated similar results on an out-patient basis although 2 cases of dural tap were encountered as predicted by Barry and Hume-Kendall[4]. The results of the present study are comparable to theirs, although by using the caudal route, patients could be managed more simply on an out-patient basis and virtually without risk of dural tap as emphasised by Cyriax[29]. Snoek *et al.*[103] and Cuckler *et al.*[28] discouraged the use of epidural steroids as a result of their studies. However, their additional admission criteria indicated that all patients had both a neurological deficit and a significant myelographic defect. Such patients could be considered to be suffering from severe sciatica, and to be less responsive to conservative management. Secondly, assessments, including determination of spinal mobility and neurological deficit took place within 1 and 3 days of the procedure. Such parameters are slow to improve and it is likely that changes may not be evident for several months. Pain, the most relevant parameter, may take up to 10 days to respond[4,91]. Thirdly, only 2 ml and 7 ml volumes of methylprednisolone injection were administered on single occasions. It is questionable whether such volumes could always reach the appropriate nerve root on a single administration. The present study employed a 25 ml injection volume which was considered sufficient to reach the L3 level when administered via the caudal route[20]. The injection was also repeated on a second occasion, 2 weeks later, on the basis of a study performed by Burn *et al.*[21].

Having demonstrated the efficacy of epidural injection in the management of sciatica, the exact means of effect is still open to debate. If one accepts that the clinical pathology is of a disc compressing a nerve root, resulting in and associated with swelling and inflammation of that root as described by Kirkaldy-Willis[66], Park *et al.*[86], McCarron *et al.*[73] and Rydevik *et al.*[92], then one can consider three possible avenues of explanation. First, it may be that the introduction of a fluid into the epidural space physically influences the relationship between the disc and the nerve root. It was suggested by Evans[37], Davidson *et al.*[31], Bhatia *et al.*[10] and Gupta *et al.*[51], that the introduction of normal saline into the epidural space may be of therapeutic benefit in its own right. This could be a possible explanation for part of the improvement seen in the untreated group. Secondly, although the anaesthetic only anaesthetizes the nerve root for a short time, this may result in a breaking of a pain cycle as described by Wall and Melzac[111]. Thirdly, the introduction of a powerful corticosteroid to the intervertebral disc/nerve root interface could be expected to reduce both nerve root inflammation and swelling[11,15,43,44,66,73,77,78,81,86,92,96]. Consequently, the precipitating factors, an increase in the pressure and the inflammation, are both influenced. It would, therefore, seem logical to repeat the epidural administration of steroid and local anaesthetic in the management of sciatica, using the degree of pain as one's criterion for when to repeat the procedure. Neurological deficit is no bar to this dictum since Hakelius[52] and Weber[114] have shown that in cases of sciatica with neurological deficit, the final neurological outcome is independent of whether decompressive surgery is performed or not. However, should the patient's pain not be controlled by a reasonable number of epidural injections, then decompressive surgery, as described by Tile[108] amongst others, or possibly chemonucleolysis[89], is indicated.

In many cases, however, repeated epidural injections dramatically improve the quality of life for patients whose symptoms and signs would otherwise only gradually improve with the natural history of the disease. Caudal epidural injection of steroid and local anaesthetic is a simple and well tolerated technique which has a significant role to play in the management of patients with sciatica. This study indicates that active intervention by caudal injection of triamcinolone acetonide plus procaine hydrochloride can improve symptoms and signs in the immediate and intermediate term and that such improvement is maintained at a year. The placebo treated patients also improved but at a much slower rate.

8. A prospective clinical study to assess the pathomorphological changes which may accompany the resolution of sciatica

Ever since Mixter and Barr[80] drew attention to rupture of the intervertebral disc as a causal factor in sciatica, there has been debate about when to intervene surgically. This is well illustrated by figures showing an almost tenfold variation in the rate of surgery[32,63]. The satisfactory clinical outcome of patients avoiding surgical decompression has been documented[52,94,114] yet few studies have addressed the pathomorphological changes which may accompany this. Saal *et al.*[95] claimed to be the first to do so in 11 cases.

In 1952, Berg[9] suggested that disc protrusions did not resolve spontaneously on the basis of repeated myelographic studies in only 3 cases. More recently Teplic and Haskin[107], using computed axial tomography (CT), were able to demonstrate the spontaneous regression of herniated nucleus pulposus in 11 cases. It was therefore decided to set up this prospective study to monitor the natural resolution of sciatica with conservative management and to evaluate the radiological changes which might accompany this. Clearly this knowledge may be important in deciding on the appropriate management of sciatica.

8.1. Patient population

165 Consecutive patients, 114 males and 51 females of average age 41 years (range 17-72), presenting to a secondary referral centre with primary sciatica, thought to be due to lumbosacral nerve root compromise, were prospectively entered into the study. The average duration of symptoms prior to admission was 4.2 months (range 1-72). All patients complained of root pain and exhibited positive root tension signs. 110 Patients (67%) had positive neurological signs. Well accepted criteria were used to make the diagnosis[29].

Neurological signs were not considered contraindications to conservative management[52,114]. Patients with symptoms of cauda equina syndrome or with signs of progressive multi-radicular involvement were investigated with a view to immediate surgery. However, all 165 patients bar 6 patients with negative scans were arguably candidates for some form of decompressive surgery on presentation. High resolution CT scans of the lumbar spine were performed at L3/4, L4/5 and L5/S1 using well established criteria[40,41,105]. Particular attention was paid to the correlation of the clinical and radiological findings.

8.2. Treatment

The serial administration of 20 ml 0.5% procaine hydrochloride in normal saline with 1 ml (40 mg) of triamcinolone acetonide in females and 2 ml (80 mg) in males, via the caudal route and on an out-patient basis was the cornerstone of conservative management[22]. These injections were given at intervals ranging from weeks to several months, depending on the patient's symptoms, signs and clinical response. When this technique proved unsuccessful the lumbar[4,35,122] or posterolateral approach (periradicular/root block injection)[3,54,65] was used under x-ray control to confirm position and thus exclude faulty technique as a reason for poor response. Patients received an average of 3 injections (range 0-8) over one year. It was felt necessary to resort to a more specific injection technique (*i.e.* under x-ray control) in 39 patients (24%). Those patients who failed to make a satisfactory response were referred for surgical decompression. The remainder were finally assessed at one year and offered a follow-up CT scan at the pathological level with a view to assisting in prognosis.

8.3. Patient re-assessment

The capacity to cope with work and leisure activities and the level of pain were specifically enquired after. A visual analogue scale (VAS) was used. Patients were also specifically examined for root tension signs and neurological status. A follow-up CT scan was performed at the pathological level, the same scanner being used for both the first and follow-up scans. The scans were reviewed by two radiologists, blinded to the names of the patients, the dates and sequence of the scans and any clinical information relating to them. Great care was taken to compare identical slices (*i.e.* taken through the same anatomical level). Particular attention was paid to the intervertebral discs: pathomorphology was identified and a visual estimate of the difference between the two scans was recorded. Although quantitative CT measurements are now available, there was no ready access to this facility when the study was commenced in 1985. Further, Stoller *et al.*[105] point out that qualitative assessment is more significant than numerical measurements.

8.4. Results

Scans failed to demonstrate pathology accounting for the symptoms and signs in 6 (4%) of the patients initially scanned and they were not re-scanned. Pathology thought to be relevant was reported at the L2/3 level in 1 patient, the L3/4 in 8 patients, the L4/5 level in 78 patients and the L5/S1 level in 83 patients.

Because of poor response to conservative therapy, 23 patients (14%) were referred for surgical decompression and not re-scanned. 17 (74%) had positive neurological signs. The remaining 142 patients had made a good clinical recovery when finally re-assessed at one year.

25 Patients (15%) did not wish to be re-scanned primarily because they considered themselves to be cured. The remaining 111 (68%) were re-scanned.

The most striking feature is that 64 of the 84 herniated/sequestrated intervertebral discs showed complete or partial resolution at 1 year, whereas only 7 of the 27 bulging discs showed any resolution at 1 year. This is highly significant (Chi-squared=20.27, $P=0.0001$). Examples of partial and complete intervertebral disc resolution are shown in Figures 2 and 3.

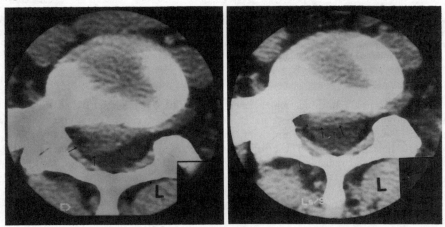

(a) (b)

Figure 2. (a) CT scan showing a substantial right posterolateral L5/S1 disc herniation in a 32 year-old male presenting with 3 months of severe lower back pain and right sciatica not responding to physiotherapy. (b) After 1 year and 2 caudal and 2 lumbar epidural injections. The patient was back to normal work, and recorded a 95% improvement in VAS pain score, SLRs were normal and both ankle jerks present and equal.

All patients re-scanned were able to work and follow their usual leisure activities. The average improvement in their level of pain on the visual analogue scale was 94% (range 45-100%) and none had root tension signs. 74 (67%) had neurological signs on presentation and, of these, 70 (95%) had made a partial or complete recovery.

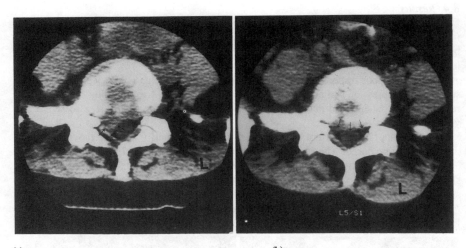

(a)   (b)

Figure 3. (a) CT scan showing a substantial right posterolateral L5/S1 disc herniation in a 27 year-old female presenting with 2 months of severe lower back pain and right sciatica not responding to bed rest and osteopathy. (b) After 1 year and 4 caudal epidural injections. The patient was back to normal work, and recorded a 100% improvement in VAS pain score, SLRs were normal but the right ankle jerk was still absent.

The important sub-groups which emerge from this study are set out in Figure 4. Between group analysis, using t-tests and chi-squared tests, was carried out on the variables to determine whether there were any significant differences between the conservatively and surgically managed groups. Those patients who required surgical decompression had a significantly greater reduction of straight leg raise ($P=0.02$) and had significantly more injections ($P=0.01$) than those who recovered with conservative management. Significantly more females underwent surgical decompression ($P=0.001$).

The categories of intervertebral disc pathomorphology can be reduced to a 2x2 table combining the categories (generalised bulge and focal bulge) versus (generalised bulge + herniation, herniation and sequestration) using individual patients rather than intervertebral discs. There is no statistically significant difference between the distribution of disc bulges and disc herniations in the conservatively or surgically managed groups (chi-squared=0.69).

Further between group analysis, using t-tests and chi-squared tests, was carried out on the variables to determine whether there were any more subtle but significant differences between the 'resolved' and 'no change' groups. Those patients whose intervertebral disc pathomorphology partially or completely resolved were significantly younger ($P=0.04$), had a shorter duration of symptoms before presentation ($P=0.01$) and had a greater reduction of SLR ($P=0.01$) than the group that showed no change.

There were no other statistically significant differences between the 'no change' and 'resolved' disc groups. However, the average improvement in pain level, on the visual analogue scale, of those patients whose discs were reported as the same or worse was 90% (range 50-100%) whereas in the patients whose discs had partly or completely resolved, it was 96% (range 45-100%). This trend is what one might have expected clinically but again was not statistically significant.

Finally, between group analysis was carried out to ascertain whether there was any significant difference between the number of injections received by males and females. Because of the occasional menstrual disturbance noted in the preliminary epidural study, females had received 40 mg of triamcinolone acetonide rather than 80 mg which was administered to the males. However, females did not require significantly more injections but significantly more eventually underwent surgical decompression.

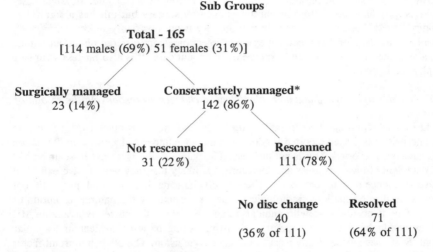

Sub Groups

Total - 165
[114 males (69%) 51 females (31%)]

Surgically managed   **Conservatively managed***
23 (14%)   142 (86%)

Not rescanned   **Rescanned**
31 (22%)   111 (78%)

No disc change   **Resolved**
40   71
(36% of 111)   (64% of 111)

*All conservatively managed patients made a good clinical recovery irrespective of radiological outcome

Figure 4. Sub-groups of patients defined by management, CT scan and whether there was an observable change in the disc.

8.5. The management of sciatica

Of patients with clinical sciatica and radiological evidence of nerve root entrapment, 86% were treated successfully by aggressive conservative management. This corresponds to the findings of Hakelius[52], Weber[114] and Saal[14] . However, there appeared to be no alternative to surgical decompression in 14% of patients. Weber[114] also found that a certain number of patients, initially allocated to conservative management, ultimately required surgical intervention. There was a high correlation between the clinical findings and the radiological evidence of nerve root compression. This corresponds with the expected sensitivity of computed tomography in the diagnosis of lumbar nerve root compression[12,40,40,55,90,106,118] and also confirms that the clinical criteria for lumbosacral nerve root compromise, applied in the preliminary study, were sound. The age and sex distribution of our series was also consistent with others[16,53,92,104,113].

These findings are in agreement with Saal[94,95] and may explain why there has been an almost ten-fold variation in the incidence of surgery between the USA and Great Britain[32,63]. Perhaps surgeons are generally less aggressive in Great Britain[32] or perhaps the length of waiting lists on the National Health Service allow sciatica to follow its natural course, despite the appeals by some surgeons for up to 55,000 operations per year rather than the present 3,000[38]. In some cases, perhaps the long waiting lists are a blessing in disguise in avoiding the trauma of surgery[32,94,104], although in others this may result in unnecessary pain and suffering. It has been possible to use the technique of epidural steroid injection, the efficacy of which has been demonstrated in previous studies[13,33,91] and confirmed[22], to make the period of natural resolution more acceptable. In some cases symptoms may have been more promptly relieved by surgery but this has a significant morbidity[32,36,88,94,104] and, rarely, mortality[104]. Surgery is not invariably successful[32,34,88,104]. Certainly an average of 3 consecutive epidural injections, administered on an out-patient basis, avoids the inconvenience and expense of in-patient care. It is also far less traumatic both physically and mentally.

8.6. The pathomorphological and pathophysiological changes accompanying the resolution of sciatica

The blinded reporting of comparable scans is self-auditing in as much as, if regression of disc herniation had been reported randomly, a higher number of increases in herniation would have been reported. This is not the case. The patients who were not re-scanned had made excellent clinical progress and therefore it is likely that they would have exhibited a similar incidence of disc regression. These results indicate that, in a high proportion of patients with disc herniations, radiological changes accompany the natural resolution of sciatica. This is not the case with annular bulges. No doubt the currently available MR facilities would be even more specific in distinguishing between nuclear and annular material. Saal[95] has independently reached the same conclusion. The other important factor in this condition is inflammation. Whilst this is undoubtedly partly due to the pressure at the intervertebral disc/nerve root interface[86,92,93], other factors such as chemical and auto-immune reactions do play a part[11,15,43,44,66,73,77,78,81,92,96]. The placement of corticosteroids around the nerve root may be expected to reduce this inflammation and the swelling and oedema[86,92,93] which accompanies this, thus partly relieving the pressure. In time, the factors precipitating the rise in pressure and inflammation may resolve. Of course, this may occur without discernable change occurring on computed tomography. This would account for the generally good progress of patients whose scans were not reported to demonstrate change, although their average pain scores were slightly higher. In any event, up to 35% of asymptomatic people have been reported to have abnormal computed tomographic scans[117]. There have also been reports of disc herniations eroding bone[64,85] and thus effectively creating more space and less pressure. The striking feature of this study is the high percentage of disc herniations which showed partial or complete resolution at one year. Perhaps this percentage and the degree of resolution would have been even greater on a longer time scale. This would seem to support the suggestion made by Cyriax[29] and suspected by many others, that herniated nuclear material "shrivels up" in time. More precisely this may be due to the gradual enzymatic degradation of the proteoglycans[83,100] and resultant loss of water content[2,39,45] with additional phagocytic activity[73,87,96] associated with neovascularisation[46].

No correlation was demonstrated between disc resolution and the final neurological outcome. However, Yates[120] points out that the return of muscular power can be accounted for by re-innervation from adjacent nerve roots, which takes place at the motor end plate.

8.7. The clinical and radiological features affecting outcome

It would seem that substantial limitation of straight leg raise and being female are predisposing factors towards surgery. The presence of neurological signs was certainly not an absolute indication for surgery[52,114]: 66% of conservatively managed patients and 74% of those undergoing surgery had neurological signs. Although there was a trend for intervertebral disc herniations (as opposed to bulges) to require surgical intervention, this was not statistically significant and indeed intervertebral disc herniations showed a highly significant predisposition towards spontaneous resolution ($P=0.0001$).

Youth and a shorter duration of symptoms were statistically in favour of intervertebral disc resolution. This was also the case for patients with a greater reduction of straight leg raise and of course those with intervertebral disc herniations (as opposed to bulges). Thus although increased limitation of straight leg raise was a statistically significant predisposing factor towards surgery, it was also a statistically significant predisposing factor towards the resolution of intervertebral disc pathomorphology.

8.7. Summary and future research

These results confirm the CT findings of Teplick and Haskin[107] on a larger scale. It has also been possible to analyze them with respect to both the clinical presentation and outcome, and thus independently reach the same conclusions as Saal et al.[95].

Taking into account the mechanisms whereby intervertebral disc herniations may resolve spontaneously[39,45,46,73,83,87,96,100] it would seem likely that this occurs when nuclear material is exposed to the environment of the epidural space. Since it is possible to differentiate further between annulus fibrosus and nucleus pulposus with magnetic resonance imaging, in the future it may be possible to predict even more precisely which intervertebral disc pathomorphology is likely to resolve spontaneously. Contemporary scanners also offer the facility for quantitative assessment. There is thus much scope for further research in this field.

9. Conclusions

Epidural corticosteroids are efficacious in the management of intractable sciatica. If inflammation and thus pain can be suitably controlled by serial epidural or periradicular corticosteroid infiltrations, then most patients suffering from intractable discogenic sciatica will recover without the need for surgical intervention.

A high proportion of intervertebral disc herniations have the potential to resolve spontaneously. Even if patients have marked reduction of straight leg raise, positive neurological signs and a substantial intervertebral disc herniation (as opposed to a bulge) there is potential for making a natural recovery, not least due to resolution of the intervertebral disc herniation. Indeed, the intervertebral disc pathomorphology which might seem best suited to surgical resection is in fact that which shows the most significant incidence of natural regression. Male patients with sciatica would seem to have a better chance of avoiding surgery than females.

Up until now it has been difficult for the clinician, faced with a patient suffering from sciatica in association with a substantial radiological defect, to answer the question: "how will I ever recover if the mechanical factor causing my sciatica is not removed?" These results confirm that if the pain can be controlled, nature can be allowed to run its course with the partial or complete resolution of the mechanical factor. Nonetheless, there is clearly always a place for surgical decompression of patients suffering from cauda equina syndrome, multi-radicular neurological deficit and when aggressive conservative management fails.

10. Acknowledgment

The research presented in this chapter forms part of a dissertation submitted to the University of London for the degree of Doctor of Medicine.

11. References

1.   S.E. Abram and R.W. Cherwenka, *Anaesthesiology* **50** (1979) 461-462.
2.   P. Adams, D.R. Eyre and H. Muir, *Rheumat. Rehab.* **16** (1977) 222-229.
3.   M. Bard and J. Laredo, *Interventional radiology in bone and joint.*Springer-Verlag Wien, New York, (1988) p.101-156.
4.   P.J.C. Barry and P. Hume Kendall, *Ann. Phys. Med.* **6** (1962) 267-273.
5.   H.K. Beard and R.C. Stevens, in *The Lumbar Spine and Backpain* 2nd edn., ed. M.I.V. Jayson (Pitman, London 1980) p. 407-436.
6.   P. Beliveau, *Rheum. Phys. Med.* **11** (1971) 40-43.
7.   G.R. Bell and R.B. Rothman, *Spine* **9** (1984) 54-56.
8.   H.T. Benzon, *Pain* **24** (1986) 277-295.
9.   A. Berg, *Acta. Chir. Scan.* **104** (1952) 124-129.
10.   M.T. Bhatia and L.C.J. Parikh, *J. Indian Med. Assoc.* **47** (1966) 537-542.
11.   P. Bobechko and C. Hirsch, *J. Bone Joint Surg.* **47B** (1965) 574-584.
12.   S.J Bosacco, A. T. Berman, J.L. Garbarino *et al.*, *Clin. Orthop.* **190** (1984) 124-128.
13.   H. Breivik, P.E. Helsa, I. Molnar *et al.*, in *Advances in Pain Research and Therapy* Vol. 1, eds. J.J. Bonica and D. AlbeFessard (Raven Press, New York, 1976) p.927-931.
14.   C. Briceno, M. Fazl, R.A. Willinsky and S. Gertzbein, *Spine* **14** (1989) 898-899.
15.   F.W.Brown, *Clin. Orthop.* **129** (1977) 72-78.
16.   I. Bruske-Hohlfeld, J.C. Merritt, B.M. Onofrio *et al.*, *Spine* **15** (1990) 31-35.

17. J.R. Bullard and F.M. Houghton, *Anesth. Analg.* **56** (1977) 862-863.
18. J.M.B. Burn and L. Langdon, *Rheumatol. Phys. Med.* **10** (1970) 368-374.
19. J.M.B. Burn, *Proc. Roy. Soc. Med.* **66** (1973) 28.
20. J.M. Burn, P.B. Guyer and L. Langdon, *Br. J. Anaesth.* **45** (1973) 338-345.
21. J.M. Burn and L. Langdon, *Am. J. Phys. Med.* **53** (1974) 29-34.
22. K. Bush and S.Hillier, *Spine* **16** (1991) 572-575.
23. M.F. Cathelin, *Soc. Biol., Paris* **53** (1901) 452-453.
24. G. Caussade and P. Queste, *Societé Médicale Des Hopitaux, Paris* **28** (1909) 865-877.
25. K.O. Cho, American Surgeon **36** (1970) 303-308.
26. E.N. Coombes, *Br. Med. J.* **1** (1961) 20-24.
27. B. Corrigan, G. Carr and S. Tugwell, *Med. J. Australia* (1982) 224-225.
28. J.M. Cuckler, P.A. Bernini, S.W. Weisel *et al.*, *J. Bone Joint Surg.* **67A** (1986) 63-66.
29. J. Cyriax, *Textbook of Orthopaedic Medicine Vol 1. Diagnosis of Soft Tissue Lesions.*8th edn., (Bailliere Tindall, London, 1984) p. 221-360.
30. P. Daly, *Anaesthesia* **25** (1970) 346-348.
31. J.T. Davidson and G.C. Robin, *Brit. J. Anaesth.* **33** (1961) 595-598.
32. R.A. Dickson, Current Orthop. **1** (1987) 387-390.
33. T.P.W. Dilke, H.C. Burry and R. Grahame, *Br. Med. J.* **2** (1973) 635-637.
34. J. Dvorak, M.H. Gauchat and L. Valach, *Spine* **13** (1988) 1416-1422.
35. I. Emery and H. Gordon, *Clin. Radiol.* **31** (1980) 643-649.
36. G. Evans and R.K. Jackson, *Br. Med. J.* **297** (1988) 5.
37. W. Evans, Lancet **2** (1930) 1225-1229.
38. A. Ferriman, One-day back operation could save NHS millions. *Observer* July 22nd (1990) p.6.
39. R. Fick, *Handbuch der Anatomie und Mechanik der Glenke.* Jena, Gustav Fisher Verlag (1904) p. 57-88.
40. H. Firooznia, V. Benjamin, I.I. Kricheff *et al.*, *Am. J. Radiol.* **142** (1984) 587-592.
41. J.W. Fries, D.A. Abodeely, Vinjungco *et al.*, *J. Comput. Assist. Tomogr.* **6** (1982) 874-887.
42. H.S. Gasser and J. Erlanger, A*mer. J. Physiol.* **88** (1929) 581-591.
43. S.D. Gertzbein, *Clin. Orthop.* **129** (1977) 68-71.
44. S.D. Gertzbein, J.H. Tait and S.R. Devlin, *Clin. Orthop.* **123** (1977) 149.
45. C. Gocke, *Arch. Orthop. Unfall. Chirurg.* **31** (1931) 42-80.
46. I. Goldie, *Acta Pathol. Scand.* **42** (1958) 302-304.
47. J. Gordon, *Anaesthesia* **35** (1980) 515-516.
48. R. Grahame, *Clinics in Rheum. Diseases* **6** (1980) 143-157.
49. P.W.B Green, A.J. Burke, C.A. Weiss, *Clin. Orthop.* **153** (1980) 121-125.
50. A.W. Grogono and D.J. Woodgate, *Lancet* (1971) 1024-1026.
51. A.K. Gupta, V.K. Mital and R.V. Azmi, *J. Indian Med. Assoc.* **54** (1970) 194-196.

52.   A. Hakelius, *Acta Orthop. Scan. (Suppl.)* **129** (1970) 1-76.
53.   B.B. Hall and J.A. McCulloch, *J. Bone Joint Surg.* **65A** (1983) 1215-1219.
54.   M. Hasue, J. Kunogi, S. Konno *et al.*, *Spine* **14**: (1989) 1261-1264.
55.   V. Haughton, O. Eldevik, B. Magnaes *et al.*, *Radiology* **142** (1982) 103-110.
56.   M. Helliwell, J.C. Robertson and R.M. Ellis, *Br. J. Clin. Pract.* **39** (1985) 228-231.
57.   G.Heyse-Moore, *Acta Orthop. Scand.* **49** (1978) 366-370.
58.   A. Iggo, in *UFAW Symposium, Assessments of Pain in Man and Animals*, eds. C.A. Keele and R. Smith (Livingstone, London, 1962) p. 74-78.
59.   R. Ito, *J. Jap. Orthop. Assoc.* **45** (1971) 769-777.
60.   D.W. Jackson, A. Rettig and L. Wiltse, *Am. J. Sports Med.* **8** (1980) 239-243.
61.   R.K. Jackson, *J. Bone Joint Surg.* **53B** (1971) 609-616.
62.   F.O. Jennings and E.J. Delaney, *Irish Med. J.* **72** (1979) 402-406.
63.   W.J Kane,The incidence rate of laminectomies. *Proceedings of the International Society for the Study of the Lumbar Spine Meeting.* New Orleans, May 1980.
64.   H. Kelman, *Am. J. Surg.* **64**(1944) 183-190.
65.   S. Kikuchi, M. Hasue, K. Nishiyama *et al.*, *Spine* **9** (1984) 23-30.
66.   W.H. Kirkaldy-Willis, *Spine* **9** (1984) 49-52.
67.   C. Klenerman, R. Greenwood, H.T Davenport *et al.*, *Br. J. Rheumatol.* **23** (1984) 35-38.
68.   C. L. Knight and J.C. Burnell, *Anaesthesia* **35** (1980) 593-594.
69.   O. Knutsen and H. Ygge, *Acta Orthop. Scand.* **42** (1971) 338-352.
70.   M.Kosteljanetz, F. Bang and S. Schmidt-Elsen, *Spine* **13** (1988) 393-395.
71.   W.Y.Loebl, *Ann. Phys. Med.* **9** (1967) 103-110.
72.   W. Luyendijk and A.E. van Voorthuisen, *Acta Radiol.* **5** (1966) 1051-1066.
73.   R.F. McCarron, M.W. Wimpee, P.G. Hudkins *et al.*, *Spine* **12** (1987) 758.
74.   P.F. McCombe, J.C.T. Fairbank, B.C. Cockersole *et al.*, *Spine* **14** (1989) 908-918.
75.   J.A.McCulloch, *Clin. Orthop.* **146** (1980) 128-135.
76.   R. MacIntosh and R. Bryce-Smith, *Local Analgesia - Abdominal Surgery*, 2nd edn., (Livinstone, Edinburgh, 1962) p. 26-31.
77.   L.L. Marshall and E.R. Trethewie, Lancet **2** (1973) p. 320.
78.   L.L. Marshall, E.R. Trethewie and C.C. Curtain, *Clin. Orthop.* **129** (1977) 61-67.
79.   J.A. Mathews and D.A.H. Yates, *Br. Med. J.* **3** (1969) 696-697.
80.   W.J. Mixter and J.S. Barr, *New Eng. J. Med.* **211** (1934) 210-215.
81.   R.W. Murphy, *Clin. Orthop.* **129** (1977) 46-60.
82.   S.E. Natelson, C.E. Gibson and R.A. Gillespie, *Southern Med. J.* **13** (1980) 286-287, 306.
83.   A. Naylor, *Orthop. Clin. North Am.* **2** (1971) 343-359.

84. D.A. Nelson, T.S. Vates and R.B. Thomas, *Acta Neurol. Scand.* **49**: (1973) 176-188.
85. J.F. Norfray, Gadom, R.C. Becker *et al.*, *Spine* **13** (1988) 941-944.
86. W.W. Parke and R.Y.O. Watanabe, *Spine* **10** (1985) 508-515.
87. J.B. Pennington, R.F. McCarron and G.S. Laros, *Spine* **13** (1988) 909-912.
88. H.C. Pheasant and P. Dyck, *Clin. Orthop.* **164** (1982) 93-109.
89. F. Postacchini, R. Lami and M. Massorbrio, *Spine* **12** (1987) 87-96.
90. S. Raskin and J. Keatin, *Am. J. Neuroradiol.* **3** (1982) 215-221.
91. M.G. Ridley, G.H. Kingsley, T. Gibson *et al.*, *Br. J. Rheumatol.* **27** (1988) 295-299.
92. B. Rydevik, M.D. Brown and G. Ludborg, *Spine* **9** (1984) 7-15.
93. B. Rydevik, R.R. Myers and H.C. Powell, *Spine* **14** (1989) 575-577.
94. J.A. Saal and J.S. Saal, *Spine* **14** (1989) 431-437.
95. J.A. Saal, J.S. Saal and R.J. Herzog, *Spine* **15** (1990) 683-686.
96. J.S. Saal, R. Sibley, R. Dobrow *et al.*, *Cellular response to lumbar disc herniation: An immuno-histologic study. Proceedings of the International Society for the Study of the Lumbar Spine Meeting.* Boston, Mass. (1990).
97. T. Sakuragi, K. Higa, K. Dan *et al.*, *The Pain Clinic* **1** (1987) 183-188.
98. W. Sayle-Creer and M. Swerdlow, *Acta Orthop. Belgica* **35** (1969) 728-734.
99. C. Sciaretta, *Clin. Therap.* **49** (1969) 269-275.
100. K.A. Sedowofia, I.W. Tomlinson, J.B. Weiss *et al.*, *Spine* **7** (1982) 213-222.
101. P.K. Sharma, *Postgraduate Med. J.* **53** (1977) 1-6.
102. A. Sicard, *Comptes Rendus Hebdomadaires des Séances et Memoires de la Societé de Biologie* **53** (1901) 396-398.
103. W. Snoek, H. Weber and B. Jorgensen, *Acta Orthop. Scand.* **48** (1977) 535.
104. E.V. Spangfort, *Acta Orthop. Scand.* **142** (1972) 1-95.
105. D.W. Stoller, H.K. Genant, N.I. Chafetz *et al.*, *Current Orthop.* **1** (1987) 219-226.
106. S. Tchang, J. Howie, W. Kirkaldy-Willis *et al.*, *J. Can. Assoc. Radiol.* **33** (1982) 15-20.
107. J.G. Teplick and M.E. Haskin, *Am. J. Neuroradiology* **6** (1985) 331-335.
108. M.Tile, *Spine* **9** (1984) p. 57-64.
109. M. Trotter, *Anesth. and Analg.* **26** (1947) 192-202.
110. G. Waddell, T.A. McCulloch, E.D. Kummel *et al.*, *Spine* **5** (1980) 117-125.
111. P. D. Wall and R. Melzack, *Textbook of Pain.* (Churchill Livingstone, London, 1984) p. 240-251.
112. A. C. Warr, J.A. Wilkinson, J.M.B. Burn *et al.*, *Practitioner* **209** (1972) 53-59.
113. H. Weber, *J. Oslo City Hosp.* **28** (1978) 33-61, 91-113.
114. H. Weber, *Spine* **8** (1983) 131-140.
115. J. Weinstein, W. Claverie and S. Gibson, *Spine* **13** (1988) 1344-1351.
116. A. H. White, R. Derby and G. Wynne, *Spine* **5** (1980) 78-86.
117. S.W. Wiesel, N. Tsourmas, H.I. Feffer *et al.*, *Spine* **9** (1984) 549-551.

118. A. Williams, V. Haughton and A. Syvertsen, *Radiol. Med. (Torino)* **135** (1980) 95-99.
119. A.P. Winnie, J T. Hartman, H.L. Meyers *et al.*, *Anaesthesia Anal. Cur. Res.* **51** (1972) 990-999.
120. D.A.H. Yates, *Ann. Phys. Med.* **7** (1964) 169-179.
121. D.W. Yates, *Rheumatol. Rehab.* **17** (1978) 181-186.
122. M. Zenz, C. Panhans, Chr. H. Niesel *et al.*, *Regional anaesthesia* (Wolfe Med. Pub. 1988) p. 106-116.

INDEX